The Holland Method™ of Advanced Reflexology

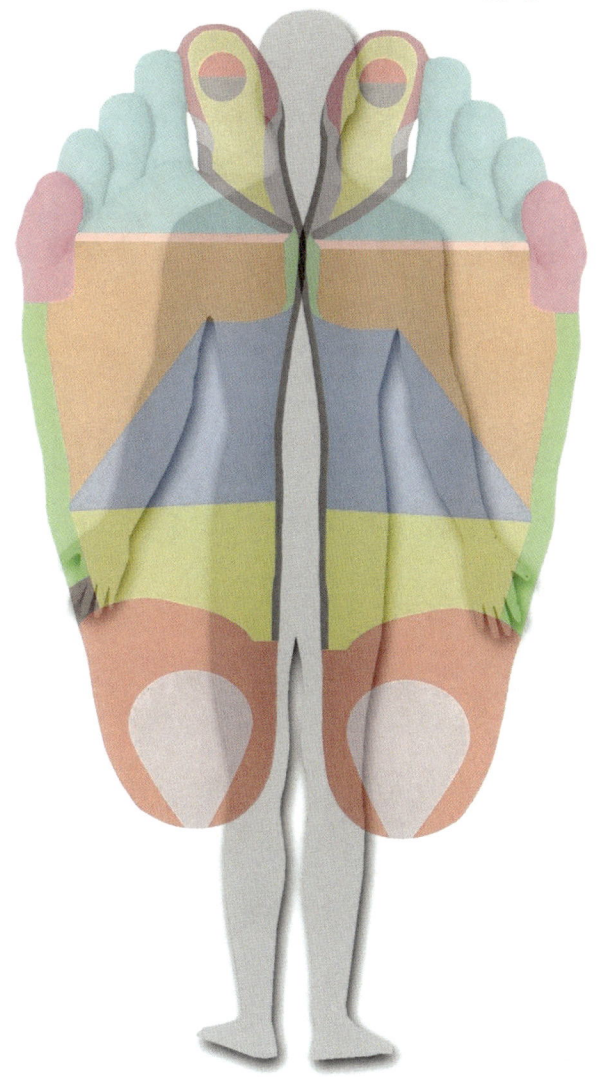

by Douglas R. Holland, Jr.

Reflexology Redefined

The Holland Method™ of Advanced Reflexology

by

Doug Holland, IR
Master Reflexologist

Andover Publishing
Andover, Ohio
www.hollandreflexology.com
United States of America

Copyright 2009 by Douglas R. Holland, Jr.

All rights reserved. No part of this book may be reproduced in any manner whatsoever without written permission from the author or Andover Publishing with the exception in the instance of a brief quotation in critical and scientific articles and reviews, with the term 'brief' defined by Douglas R. Holland, Jr.

This book or parts of it may not be used for teaching, class instruction or educational seminars outside of those given by The Holland Institute of Advanced Reflexology. This book is licensed solely for individual use by a single owner for his or her personal instruction and reference in conducting his or her own practice. Any other use will be considered 'infringement of copyright'.

Acknowledgments

I am grateful for the help of my family in putting this book together:

My wife, Lori, who helped write, edit and create the graphics and photos for this book.

I'd like to thank my son, Bo, and my daughter, Paige, for patiently modeling for me for the images and being quiet when I needed to think!

Thanks to my mother-in-law, Lina Simmons, for editing this book.

Much appreciation to Harold Charleston and his wife, Gail, for their continued support.

I'd also like to thank Dr. Patricia Lawson, Director of Clinical Integrative Certification Programs.

Foreword

When I learned reflexology and started practicing it, I felt a sense of purpose, because 1) I knew I am a good reflexologist and going to get better every day and 2) because I knew I was really helping people. But helping several people daily isn't enough. I am convinced that the more people that know about this practice and try to learn it, the better we'll all be, health-wise.

It is my hope in writing this book that I can help foster, nurture and encourage an interest in learning and performing the art of reflexology. I am not a medical doctor but I am an Integrative Reflexologist and feel strongly that reflexology deserves its place amongst the modalities that make up Integrative Medicine.

With the learning and research I have done, as well as writing my own findings, I am still continuing my journey learning and discovering about reflexology. I plan on doing that until the day I die! It is my wish that I help set you, the reader, on your own journey to learn and practice this wonderful modality.

*A note to students and readers: Because of my dyslexia, I have added phonetic spellings in places throughout the book that are not the 'dictionary' phonetic spellings with proper diacritics but spellings that **I** can understand; as I have difficulty in remembering proper pronunciation of the Latin-based language. Hopefully they won't be too distracting for you.*

Table of Contents

1	**The History of Reflexology**..	1
2	**What is the Holland Method of Reflexology?**.............................	5
	Explanation..	6
	What is a Reflex?..	7
	Thumb-driving...	8
	What Creates a Pulse...	8
	Observation & Pain..	11
	Why Intense Pain is Felt When Abnormalities are Found........	12
	Can All Benefit From Reflexology?...	13
	Human Touch is Superior to Fabricated Tools.........................	14
	Do Reflexes Reveal Specific Sickness?....................................	14
	How to Handle Our Observations...	15
	Traditional Charts and Diagnosis..	15
	Dominant Theory vs. Zone Theory..	16
	Contradictions in Pain...	18
	Hierarchal Pain Leads to New Understandings........................	18
	Reflex Table Chart..	20
	Systems Involved with Communication....................................	21
	Powerful Tools to Unlock Communication................................	21
	How the Body Can Mask Pain to Defend Itself.........................	22
	To Diagnose or Not to Diagnose?...	23
	The Three Types of Congestion..	24
	Why Communicate Anything to The Client?.............................	25
	The Priority Level of Reflexology..	25
3	**The Anatomy of the Feet**...	29
	Foot Basics...	30
	Look at the Bones..	31
	The Arches...	32

3	Pronation	33
	Supination	34
	Muscles of the Feet	34
	Tendons of the Feet	35
	Nerves of the Feet	35
4	**Conditions That Can Affect the Feet**	**37**
	Arthritis	38
	Gout	38
	Osteoarthritis	39
	Rheumatoid Arthritis	39
	Tarsal Tunnel Syndrome	39
	Calluses	40
	Corns	40
	Diabetes and the Foot	41
	Neuropathy	41
	Poor Circulation	42
	Plantar Fasciitis	42
	What is Plantar Fascia?	43
	Heel Spur	43
	Metatarsalgia	44
	Achilles' Tendonitis	45
	Athlete's Foot	45
	Dry Skin	46
	Clubfoot	46
5	**Conditions of the Toes**	**47**
	Claw Toes	48
	Mallet Toes	49
	Hammer Toes	49
	Morton's Toe	50
	Bunions	50
	Webbed Toes	51

5	Toenail Fungus	52
	Ingrown Toenails	53
6	**Understanding the Charts**	55
	Guidelines for the Holland Method Chart	57
	The Holland Method of Reflexology Chart (plantar view)	60
	The Holland Method of Reflexology Chart (medial & lateral views)	61
	The Dominant Reflex Chart	62
	The Intermedial Reflex Chart	63
7	**Taking Care of Yourself and Your Equipment**	65
	Dorsal Flexing	66
	Plantar Flexing	67
	Adduction Wrist Stretch	67
	Abduction Wrist Stretch	67
	Phalanges Exercise	68
	Keep Your Nails Trimmed	68
	Halitosis	69
	Cleanliness	69
	Colognes	70
	Equipment	70
	Music	71
	Lighting	71
8	**Thumb-driving, Holding, Stretching and Relaxation Techniques**	73
	Thumb-driving (walking)	74
	Basic Finger Techniques	75
	Length of Treatment	76
	Levels of Pressure	77
	• Level One	77
	• Level Two	77
	• Level Three	78
	How to Gain Proper Leverage with the Holding Hand	79

8   Holding.. 80
       Stretching... 80
       Tarsal Stretch.. 80
       Metatarsal Stretching... 81
- Adduction.. 82
- Abduction.. 82

       Metatarsal Wrenching... 82
       Digital Dorsal Flexing and Achilles Stretching..................................... 84
       Relaxation Techniques.. 85
       Calcaneus Rocking.. 85
       Hand Drill.. 86
       Metatarsal Wave.. 87
       Hanging the Saddle... 88

9   **Getting Ready to Administer a Reflexology Treatment**.................... 91
       Preparing Mentally for Client & Greeting.. 92
       Greeting: At First Sight.. 93
       Intent Statement Explained.. 94
       Be Careful of What You Say.. 95
       Oils & Lotions.. 96
       Beginning Treatment.. 96

10   **Hierarchal Treatment: The Dominant Reflexes**................................. 99
       The Amygdala / Brain Reflex – The Most Dominant Reflex............... 100
       The Brain.. 103
       Performing the Amygdala / Brain Reflex... 104
       The Hypothalamus Reflex – The Second Most Dominant Reflex....... 106
       Pituitary / Pineal – The Third Most Dominant Reflex......................... 107
       The Pineal Gland.. 108
       Performing the Hypothalamus / Pituitary / Pineal Reflex Technique.. 109
       Trapezius Shoulders – The Fourth Most Dominant Reflex................. 110
       Performing the Trapezius Shoulders Reflex.. 112
- Walking the Ridge... 112

10	• Plantar Digits Down	114
	• Plantar Digits Up	114
	• Dorsal Digits Down	115
	The Hip / Sciatic – The Fifth Most Dominant Reflex	116
	Performing the Hip / Sciatic Reflex	118
	• Medial Compression & Extension	118
	• Lateral Compression & Extension	118
	• Medial Finger Drive	119
	• Lateral Finger Drive	119
	• Thumb-walking of the Plantar Pad	120
	The Spine – The Sixth and Last of the Dominant Reflexes	121
	Effects of Spinal Misalignments Table Chart	124
	Performing the Spine Reflex	125
11	**Hierarchal Treatment: The Intermedial Reflexes**	**129**
	Occipitalis – The Alpha of the Intermedial Reflexes	130
	Performing the Occipitalis Reflexes	131
	Sternocleidomastoid / Neck – The Second of the Intermedial Reflexes	132
	Performing the Sternocleidomastoid / Neck Reflexes	132
	Thyroid / Parathyroid – The Second of the Intermedial Reflexes	134
	The Parathyroid Glands	135
	Performing the Thyroid / Parathyroid Reflexes	136
	Adrenals – The Fourth of the Intermedial Reflexes	138
	Performing the Adrenal Reflexes	13
	Pancreas – The Fifth of the Intermedial Reflexes	139
	Performing the Pancreatic Reflexes	140
	Liver – The Sixth of the Intermedial Reflexes	141
	Performing the Liver Reflexes	142
	Kidneys – The Seventh of the Intermedial Reflexes	143
	Performing the Kidneys Reflex	144
12	**Hierarchal Treatment: The Elementary Reflexes**	**145**
	Sinus, Head, Eyes & Ears Reflexes	147

12
- Sinus 147
  - Head 147
  - Eyes 148
  - Ears 148

Performing the Sinus, Head, Eyes & Ears Reflexes 150

The Heart, Pectoralis Major, Ribs, Esophagus, Bronchial, Breasts Reflexes ... 151
- The Heart 151
- The Pectoralis Major 152
- The Ribs 152
- The Esophagus 153
- The Bronchials 153
- The Breasts 154

Performing the Heart, Pectoralis Major, Ribs, Esophagus, Bronchial, Breasts Reflexes 154

The Deltoids Reflex 155

Performing the Deltoids Reflex 155

The Stomach Reflex 156

Performing the Stomach Reflex 156

The Gallbladder Reflex 158

Performing the Gallbladder Reflex 158

The Spleen Reflex 158

Performing the Spleen Reflex 158

The Arms, Hands, Elbows, Wrist, Biceps, Triceps Reflexes 159

Performing the Arms, Hands, Elbows, Wrist, Biceps, Triceps Reflexes ... 159

The Small Intestine, Colon, Bladder, Ureters, Testes, Ovaries, Uterus, Prostate Reflexes 160
- Small Intestine 160
- Colon 160
- Bladder 161
- Ureters 161
- Testes 161
- Prostate 161
- Ovaries 162

| 12 | • Uterus | 162 |

Performing the Colon, Small Intestines, Bladder, Ureters, Testes, Ovaries, Uterus, Prostate Reflexes 163

Ileocecal Valve / Appendix Reflexes 164

Performing the Ileocecal Valve / Appendix Reflexes 164

The Legs, Knees, Achilles Tendons, Gastrocnemius, Hamstrings, Quadriceps Reflexes 165

- Legs 165
- Knees 165
- Achilles Tendon 166
- Gastrocnemius 167
- Hamstrings 167
- Quadriceps 167

Performing the Legs, Knees, Achilles Tendons, Gastrocnemius, Hamstrings, Quadriceps Reflexes 167

The Clavicles Reflex 168

Performing the Clavicles Reflex 168

The Sternum Reflex 169

Performing the Sternum Reflex 169

The Latissimus Dorsi Reflex 170

Performing the Latissimus Dorsi Reflex 170

The Gluteus Maximus / Low Back Reflexes 171

Performing the Gluteus Maximus / Low Back Reflexes 171

13 The Lymphatic System 173

14 Observations 177

A Physician's Experience with Reflexology 178

Menstrual Irregularities 180

Stroke Victim 183

Painful Feet at Work 185

Pain in the Feet When a Loved One Dies 185

Infertility Helped By Reflexology Treatments 186

Reflexology Helps Hip and Knee Pain 187

15	**Business & Ethics**...	189
	Scheduling..	190
	Fees...	191
	File System..	192
	Insurances..	193
	Associations..	193
	Ethics...	194
	General Terms...	197
	Index..	199
	Bibliography...	207
	About the Author..	208

Chapter One

The History of Reflexology

Chapter 1 – The History of Reflexology

From Where and When Did Reflexology Spring?

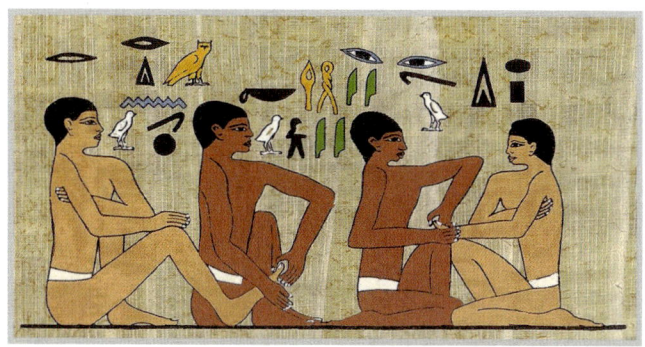

Throughout world history there are fragmented hieroglyphs of individuals who appear to be pressing on points of the feet and hands (or who may be looking to the feet and hands) to help with pain and sickness as well as other diseases. These hard-to-discern pieces of archeology point to possibilities that the feet or hands had some profound aspect on one's health or were staples in general well-being. Some of these hieroglyphic recordings may go back as far as five thousand years ago.

One example is an Egyptian hieroglyph from approximately 2330 B.C., used repeatedly in various reflexology publications and studies, that some say is the clearest expression of a possible pressure treatment to the feet and hands. This pictograph is from an Egyptian tomb (known as 'The Physician's Tomb') that depicts four persons with one appearing to be treated with pressure to the foot and another with pressure to the hand.

Other examples through the ages include: Doctors Adamus and A'Tatis and later Dr. Ball who published medical dissertations in the 16th century on zone therapy. Benvenuto Cellini (1500-1571) was known as a great Florentine sculptor who used acupressure on his fingers and toes; as well as American President James A. Garfield (1831-1881) who used the applying of pressure on the feet to relieve pain.

The individual who deserves credit for trying to bring structure and understanding to how these pressure points may work is Dr. William Fitzgerald. Born in 1872 in Connecticut, he graduated in medicine from the University of Vermont in 1895. Pursuing his career in Vienna, Austria, he came across the work of Dr. H. Bressler who had, himself, researched why pressure points on the feet may affect organs of the body, publishing these findings in <u>Zone Therapy</u>. Dr. Fitzgerald applied these techniques to his patients with the aids of rubber bands, combs, clamps and other implements.

Through his work he discovered that pressure in some areas of the foot would relieve pain in other specific parts of the body. In time, he decided to map the feet into ten energy zones: five portioned to the right side of the body and five to the left. These imaginary longitudinal lines appear vertically over the anatomical position of the human anatomy. These zones are drawn between the toes and fingers and divided equally to the top of the head.

This theory caught the attention of Dr. Edwin Bowers, a medical critic and writer, who originally investigated Dr. Fitzgerald's claims putting his findings to the test with individuals. His skepticism appeased, he aided Dr. Fitzgerald in developing this therapy. Dr. Fitzgerald and Dr. Edwin Bowers together published in 1917 the book <u>Zone Therapy</u>, the name by which reflexology was known until the early 1960's.

The theory was not well received by the medical community of his day but one colleague took special note; Joseph Shelby Riley, who was also a physician. Dr. Riley and his wife (yet another doctor) took Fitzgerald's courses on zone therapy to utilize in their own medical practice.

Dr. Riley's assistant just so happened to be one Eunice Ingham (1879-1974), well-known as the "Mother of Modern Reflexology." She started what we know as 'reflexology' today and she dedicated her life to researching how the reflexes and energy zones in the feet and hands correlated with the anatomical structure of the body. She also found that in the detection and response to aid in healing of the physiology of the body, the feet are more superior than the hands. As she developed her science, she wrote two books, <u>Stories The Feet Can Tell</u> and <u>Stories The Feet Have Told</u>.

This influenced one of her students, Doreen Bayley, to bring reflexology to Great Britain and the rest of Europe. Reflexology progressed since the 1960's in the United States because of others (like Dwight Byers, nephew of the late Eunice Ingham) who had taken her work seriously and continued in the development and teaching of Eunice Ingham's Method.

Other reflexologists the world over have developed their own theory through practical and scientific experience while perfecting their own art of where they believe the reflexes lie and how they affect the physiology of the body.

Chapter 1 – The History of Reflexology

Starting in 2006, we have seen such advanced theories as the Hierarchal teaching in the Dominant Theory™ of the Holland Method™ of Advanced Reflexology that I, Douglas Holland, developed. This method is a new understanding of how reflexes work and is to be differentiated from the renown theory of zone therapy. It is, I believe, the next iteration of the art and science of reflexology. Regardless, reflexology science, understanding and practice are growing exponentially and the next few years should hopefully yield the scientific proof needed for acceptance outside the holistic community.

Chapter Two

What is Reflexology?

What is Reflexology?

Reflexology is the unique modality that uses pressure from the thumb and fingers to strike reflexes in the feet that detect congestion, unlock and reopen communication and impart the need for responsible action of all body members to reach homeostasis.

The theory is that due to tension, toxins and stress, individual organs, glands and parts of the body either lose contact with superior vitals, or build up defense mechanisms that hinder normalization and good health. The goal of the reflexologist is to find and unblock congestion and re-establish communication among wayward members to achieve homeostasis.

"It's an external way to the internal way" – Doug Holland

What is the Holland Method™ of Advanced Reflexology?

The Holland Method™ of Advanced Reflexology is the method I developed through advanced studies. Based on years of experience (since 2001) I have compiled new understandings of where I believe the reflexes lie and how congestion truly interferes with healing and homeostasis. The developmental phases of my method will continue as I discover and learn new techniques.

What is unique about this method of reflexology?

- High pressure and friction from the skilled use of the thumb and forefingers to the feet increase the nonlinear communicative reflex pulse that lies within the neurophysical system.
- The "Dominant Theory™" is that the striking of dominant reflexes opens the way for intermedial and elementary reflexes to respond. Reflexes are not found in 'traditional zones' (as in Zone Therapy).
- A foot chart designed to show the reflexes in a more 'superficial anatomical' position without zones.
- Every aspect of the foot must be worked diligently to unlock as many reflexes as possible so that troubled issues can

receive the needed attention from the brain.
- More attention goes into finding and exposing problems to obtain internal healing than external relaxation techniques.
- Greater emphasis on stretching tendons, ligaments, muscles and loosening joint structures. This would include new ways to stretch and rotate the great toe, the metatarsals, the phalangeal bones and how to separate, through extension and rotation, the seven major bones of the foot. With better circulation and flexibility the reflexes can now come to the fore and be executable because the reflexologist's fingers can activate them. Light touch alone does not activate reflexes.
- The understanding that reflexes achieve peak response after several passes in a 10-12 minute time period but can be reversed (or agitated) by prolonged treatment pressure. Example: the common back scratch. The first few scratches are heavenly, the next few 'feel good' and after a short while the scratching in the same spot will start to hurt or sting from over stimulation. Reflexes are the same.
- Desire to teach basic thumb / finger techniques but allow for practitioner to develop his own art of movement. Each practitioner will have unique gifts in exposing and striking reflexes.
- Greater emphasis on the dorsal aspect of the foot.

What is a reflex as defined by the Holland Theory of Reflexology?

Before I can tell you what a reflex is, I must first lay the foundation on the fundamental understanding of the layers of the skin.

The skin has three layers: (1) **epidermis** attached by a thin membrane to the (2) **dermis**, which lies over the (3) **subcutis** (sub-**kyoo**-tis) or hypodermis. These layers are not formed together like three sheets of paper ready for a binder. Under a microscope the three different layers of skin are not attached by smooth surfaces but rather hills, valleys, nooks and crannies, square modules, round modules, etc. There seems to be no discernible

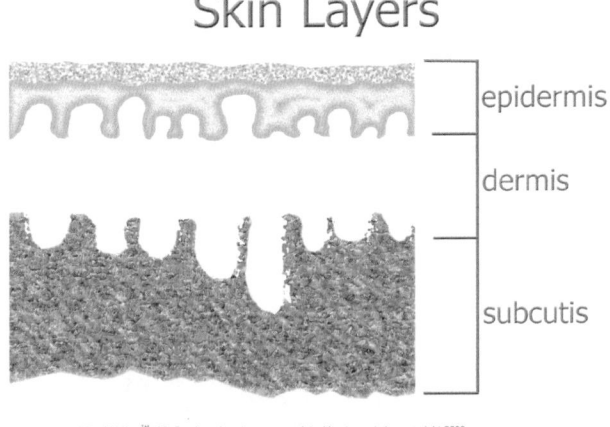

pattern to skin so it cannot loosen itself and form tears. This is why <u>thumb pressure and elongation of the skin</u> is needed to perform a reflex. How is this to be understood?

In order to create and reach a reflex these layers need to be penetrated and elongated over a specified area. The thumb and fingers travel in multiple directions over the planar surfaces of the foot. The depth in which the most distal aspect of the thumb's / finger's penetration into the dermis, epidermis and subcutis layers charges the reflex.
Imagine taking a wrinkled sheet of paper and doing your utmost to straighten and flatten it out. We're doing the same thing at the subcutaneous level of the skin. We want to remove the hills, valleys, nooks and crannies (to the best of our ability) for a brief moment in a rapid, purposeful motion.

Thumb-driving to reach reflexes

To illustrate my point of thumb pressure and elongation of the skin needed to strike a reflex, think of the sewing needle example:

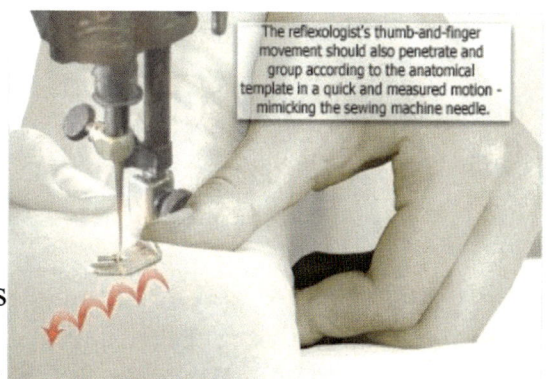

When creating this illustration, I hoped to convey the speed and movement needed to successfully reach reflexes. Look to the sewing machine and its mechanics for guidance. The machine moves the needle quickly in a measured motion - penetrating the material and connecting groupings according to a template.

The reflexologist's thumb-and-finger movement should also penetrate and group according to the anatomical template in a quick and measured motion. If the needle goes too deep, or not deep enough, or runs out of thread, or if it moves too fast or too slow, the result would be unsatisfactory. Likewise, the practitioner must use the correct amount of pressure, timing, speed and distance over the surface of the foot to satisfactorily reach the reflexes. The combinations are endless.

Grouping of nerve cells creates a pulse to the brain.

It is my opinion that a reflex formation and activation stems from the action of pushing and passing on multiple nerve cells over a specified area, from two minor anatomical points in the feet. When these two linear points come together (begin and end) from the walking pressure of the thumb over the surface of the skin, a reflex reaction occurs sending out an internal pulse asking the brain to perform a diagnostic of a specific area. This pulse travels inside the normal nervous system and dominates the brain's attention

Chapter 2 – What is Reflexology?

for a brief moment.

Intersecting points can be found and executed in thousands of different ways. In some cases, crossing large sections of the feet will yield peak reflex stimulation. Sometimes, the quicker the two points come together coupled with adequate pressure - the greater the intensity of reflex pulse (like a loud scream to the brain from the nervous system).

This special precedence, while not fully understood, is limited to the nervous system. I believe that reflexes are strong nerve cell communication at the highest level from the external to the internal.

Many of our basic functions are performed without conscious control. It becomes external when we are alerted through pain from the central nervous system - because pain cannot be ignored when an issue is in its acute state.

Pain is the brain's way to say 'something is wrong' and alert oneself that an issue has been identified through its internal diagnostics and may ask for external aid to confirm, rectify or diagnose. It's like the brain is really saying, 'Hey, if I could handle this problem myself I would not be troubling you with pain! Would you help me, for crying-out-loud?'

Pain will cause you to ask yourself to give a visual check, move, smell, feel or touch an area of concern, in order to assist in healing. How long will it take to lift up your pant leg to see what's biting you? Or how often do you flap your arms each day because of the nagging pains in the shoulder? Do you hold your crutches tightly, with each step, to protect that newly-sprained ankle?

However, we as reflexologists turn the table on the brain and force it to listen to us through the striking of reflexes during a reflexology session. The reflex pulse asks the brain to take a look at a specific area of the body and inform us if something is wrong in the form of pain. To understand this further we must first get a basic understanding of how nerves work.

The human brain contains roughly one trillion neurons, linked with up to ten thousand synaptic connections each. These neurons communicate with one another by means of long, protoplasmic fibers called **axons (axe-**sons), which carry trains of signal pulses called **action potentials** to distant parts of the brain or body and target them to specific recipient cells.

The action potential is a self-regenerating wave of electrochemical activity that allows nerve cells to carry a signal over a distance. It is the primary electrical signal generated by these action potentials (also known as **nerve impulses**) that are pulse-like waves of voltage that travel along cell membranes. These cells are the life of the body.

However, they are so tremendously complex, neurobiologists can spend their entire life on one function and still not truly understand it. I certainly don't. What we do know is that they work and work well for the entire body's association.

One example of how nerves communicate is what I call 'pain and observation'. If you touch something hot, within a picosecond, communication takes place between the sensory nerve of the epidermis and the brain and an involuntary reaction at the highest level occurs (both a motor and sensory to the brain reaction).

This reaction will take precedence over all other responsibilities of the human body during its current state of activity. How long will it take the individual to take their hand off the hot object and recognize its danger? Notice how the brain gives precedence to the crisis? If the individual does not remove his hand, serious bodily damage will occur.

You have to look at it this way; this involves two reactions. There is a reaction BEFORE a reaction. One is without conscious control (the physical reflex of taking the hand off the stove because of pain) and the other is observation of the crisis (noticing the hot stove with a quick snap of the head).

Both are closely related and occur almost simultaneously, so it is really hard to separate them into two reactions, but they are separate. The reason being is that if you had to wait until your brain processed the full consequences before it would order the emergency movement of the hand, it could be too late and bring harm to your flesh.

Some of our reflexive pain is ahead of the full internal diagnostic route. But as a rule, the internal diagnostic route is needed for resolving the issue.

Look at it from this angle: Pain is actually felt in the brain, right? So if the brain acknowledged the pain of touching the hot stove, what came first? The reaction or the

Chapter 2 – What is Reflexology?

observation? Obviously the reaction comes first under crisis (intense pain = run away first, then look). Then, through observation, which is done externally with the eyes and internally at the dermis and nerve level.

Once the alarm bell has rung, remedies can continue for the protection of the individual or the correction of the condition. In this case, fluid and nutrients will be sent to the finger to heal the wound while the individual will cognitively apply ice (cryotherapy) to reduce swelling.

However, the striking of reflexes in the feet <u>reverses</u> this entire system. Instead of 'pain and observation' which is its normal route, it becomes 'observation and pain'.

Observation and Pain

Again, the reflex pulse asks the brain for an observation of a specific area of the body in a powerful and unique way and if a problem exists (congestion or other abnormalities) pain is felt at the reflex point of contact where the thumb and fingers are working.

The pain that some clients feel when you strike a reflex can be akin to burning, stabbing, cutting or electrocution as they reflexively pull their foot back (the involuntary motor response). So often the client will ask you, 'What in the world was that?!' as they jerk their foot. Notice how the brain responds to the reflex stimuli. The greater the congestion or the finding of a new issue increases the pain. Increased pressure from the practitioner can find multiple reflexes at once causing even more pain if multiple issues reside. It is as if we are screaming at the brain and it screams back.

I believe that reflexes, with regards to reflexology, are created and are made manifest to override the nervous system to pay special attention to what the reflexes are asking for. This special attention brings about two results:

1. If there is <u>no</u> congestion or anomaly in the corresponding reflex area of the foot to the anatomical referral area, then all is well.
2. So too, when the groupings of nerve cells send out a pulse to the brain for the referral area (and back) and congestion is detected, pain is felt at the reflex point. This is to get the attention for further diagnostic processing of the brain in the strongest of manners. Then, healing can begin.

Chapter 2 – What is Reflexology?

Why is the pain felt so intensely in the feet when abnormalities are found?

For whatever reason, the body was created with backup systems that reside outside its normal function. Others are needed to assist their fellowmen in reaching these systems. Can you think of some basic needs that the body has that are revealed, revived and nurtured so that a person can be whole again?

Psychologists, among the many other modalities, come to mind. When the body is unable to help itself, others are called to aid it. The psychologist does his best to reboot the brain of a depressed soul using his own mental skill. Many treatments are usually needed. Yet, people become well again from the consoling and healing words of their practitioner. And, interestingly enough, there is no touch involved for the de-stressing of the body and yet it happens during those treatments.

But what if the psychologist skipped all the basic tools he needed to open up the patient and get them to reveal the heart of the issue, by just asking, "So what's the problem?" He would get nowhere, because if the patient knew that, they wouldn't need to sit on the couch talking to a psychologist in the first place. The response would be defensive from the beginning. Reflexes can behave the same way. They need to be systematically found, and revealed through a hierarchal system.

My theory is that passing over a dominant reflex opens the way for intermedial and elementary exposure. Sometimes a skilled reflexologist opens and strikes, in one sweeping motion, all three types of reflexes causing a powerful reaction and pulse that cannot be ignored by the brain. But we'll get into that later.

Like other modalities that naturally help people, reflexology has been around for thousands of years to do just the same - aid. And, it appears that some individuals who are interested in preventive holistic measures, use these additional tools of the system to their advantage. Therefore, to the best of my knowledge, the <u>feet were the body's designate</u> for keeping the homeostasis of oneself in check when other communications seem to have waned. And it's not hard for us to fathom this, is it? Have you ever written a note to yourself to remind you of an impending appointment the next day, only to walk right out the door the following morning, blindly missing its purpose?

Reflexes are very loud reminders to the brain to take a look around and reply back to us.

Intense pain acknowledges the need for a rebooting or clearing of a subsection of our physiology. Whatever the means, these nerves truly communicate the need to break up the congestion, reopen the channels, and promote normalization. We know that this system of checks and balances exists (the proof is in the field), and many complementary nerve cells continue to lie in wait to perform this function on our behalf.

Can all benefit from reflexology?

In my opinion, individuals with paralysis from a neck injury (severed spine) are unable to benefit from this natural diagnostic through the central nervous system. It's quite simple: They do not receive the reflex response in the form of pain nor can the brain receive the instruction to override and give precedence to the reflexologist's pressure.

I believe that clients who receive the greatest benefit from reflexology must have the central nervous system and its diagnostics intact to achieve homeostasis. This would not be the case for stroke victims. They still have the spinal column and thus the stimulation of nerves through reflexes make rehabilitation possible.

If somebody has paralysis of the legs because of a severed spine, then the hands would bring the greatest benefit for the relaxation of the client. However, I do not believe the hands can act as an internal diagnostic tool, like the feet, which reflect the needed correction by the brain to its members. The hands do have a few meaningful pressure points, but do not hold a candle to the thousands of powerful pulses that can be generated and struck in the feet which are needed for normalization.

A question I receive from time to time is: *"are you sure clients with paralysis do not receive the same benefits as those with the whole spine intact?"*

No matter how many reflexology sessions are given, once the foot is gone, it'll never grow back. Believe me, I wish I could have found proof otherwise, but in all the cases I have worked with individuals with this condition the response has been negative. The same has been the case with my ALS (Lou Gehrig's Disease) clients. As their nerves die in the feet and legs, so do the benefits.

Remember, reflexology is not a panacea or cure-all. We work with what we've got and that's it.

As a reflexologist I have seen my work transform lives and, conversely, have seen it have no impact on others. The range of outcome responses is as unique as the individuals themselves.

Human touch is superior to fabricated 'tools'.

Why is it when you're stressed and feeling down and someone gently lays a hand on your shoulder, you feel immediate release / relief? Why is human touch so comforting? Try taking a stick and touch the shoulder of a depressed soul and watch the opposite reaction.

Remember, the job of the reflex is to detect congestion, unlock and reopen communication and impart the need for responsible action of all vital members. Client pain identifies the congestion of a body member or surrounding areas by the brain.

Those members may not want to let go of their defensive stance or wake up from their sleep. Initially, repeated reflex strikes lessen client pain as the vitals become subservient to the brain's wishes and the hands of the practitioner. Reflexologists call this method simply 'working it out' - meaning working out the recalcitrant member and / or its surroundings.

After a more in depth observation (hours after the treatment) the brain will continue to stimulate these body members to get in harmony with the rest of the body.

Do reflexes always reveal specific sicknesses?

Reflexes DO NOT necessarily reveal sickness in a specified organ, gland or body part. If that was the case we, as reflexologists, could diagnose. However, since it is impossible to diagnose specific illness or maladies from the feet, reflexologists should never attempt it.

Could you diagnose a client as to having fungus in the duodenum (**doo**-uh-**dee**-num) of the small intestine, or diverticulitis of the large colon? Of course not!

People see through the falsehood when a practitioner skillfully gleans information from clients through questions and carefully works their way over to the reflex, claiming credit for the discovery when pain is induced.

But I see nothing wrong with conversing about reflex responses and how they might correlate to general issues of physiology. That's how we learn how reflexes might work.

Just be prepared to tell the client that our work helps identify congestion in those areas as we refer to the anatomical chart, and does not mean in anyway that there is an acute problem there. This is science and the charts continue to evolve; I will later expound on this in detail.

Our work is to expose imbalances only, relieve tension and stress, and reopen the lines of communication (like clearing the cobwebs) necessary for good health among the entire body's association. We assist the brain to <u>diagnose from within</u> and that is where it ends for us. A skillful reflexologist can artfully make the most stressed-out individual relax if they use the Dominant Reflex Method™.

How to handle our observations.

"But isn't there a possibility we may cause harm to the client by not revealing an important diagnosis when we feel strongly that there is merit for such alarm?"

Upon uncovering pain in a specific reflex, why can't the reflexologist make a claim for a diagnosis for a specific organ, gland or body part malfunctioning? I've worked on individuals where every reflex in the foot hurts. Does this mean that every bodily function is wrong with the client? No, that's ridiculous. However, looking at the intensity of the overall reflexes while using very minor pressure shows a lack of good general health. As a person receives a reflex session their body and all of its aspects (as a whole) begins to work together to heal its entire association, resulting in better health.

Why would traditional charts possibly mislead the client and the practitioner to make a diagnosis?

During my early reflexology career I would strike a reflex based on a traditional chart. After parroting the reflex to the client to see if he or she has an 'issue' that corresponds to that reflex or in the vertical anatomical zone - more often than not, the client would say, 'No'.

I quickly grew tired of opening up a Pandora's box of non-related problems that would then have the client nervous that something new was going on. You will learn how to ask, or glean the scientific information you desire without alarming the client. It just takes time and practice.

In my opinion, one of the greatest offenders in the vast majority of charts is the sinus reflexes being found in the toes (digits two through five). It has been my experience that the sinus reflexes are not found in the toes. Anatomically this would be logical, for if both great toes put together represents the head, then digits two through five should represent the trapezius / deltoid / shoulder conjunction. After asking clients repeatedly if this matched their feelings and symptoms, it has been deemed more accurate.

That is why I created my own anatomical chart. Not that it is dogmatically correct in every aspect but rather, a truer mirror of the entire body and the reflex association through my experience and study.

The only problem that keeps rearing its ugly head is why some reflexes seem to hurt on every visit. And some consistently hurt more than others.

What is the argument for the 'Dominant Theory™' Vs 'Zone Theory' according to the Holland Method of Reflexology?

Here is my theory of how reflexology works and it is an opinion based on working on thousands of feet since 2001. Long lasting comfort and circulation by de-stressing will not be achieved unless the 'dominant reflex' is struck with intensity.

With the dominant reflexes opened by the brain and nervous system, subservient reflexes become available for diagnosis and unlocking by the brain. How so? I will try to illustrate: A massage therapist may give 'feathers' (or light touch) to a client and achieve a measure of relaxation, however, the benefit will be short-lived because the root cause may not have been addressed.

For instance, trigger point therapy is used to remove knotted muscles which can be a painful process but the end result is deep relaxation for the muscular system. The root cause of tension was the knotted

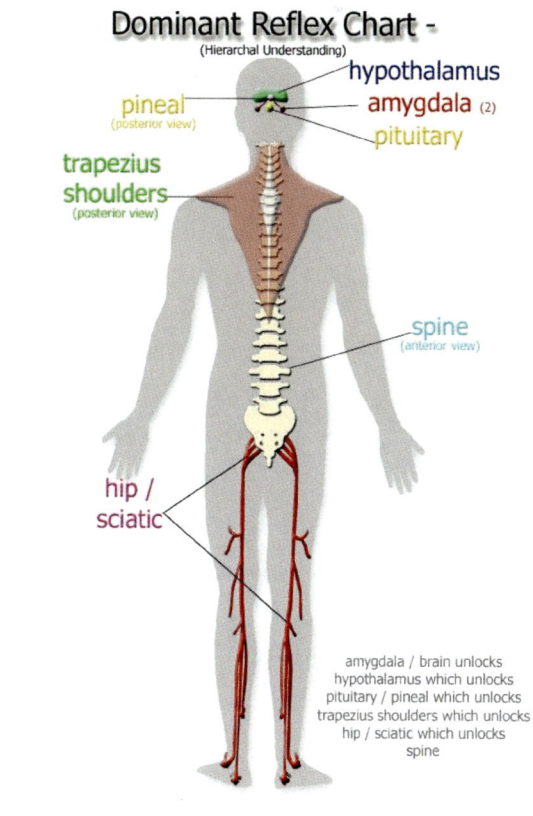

Chapter 2 – What is Reflexology?

muscle. Gentle, light touch would not have resolved that issue. A reflexologist, also, must use pressure to unlock dominant, intermedial and elementary reflexes according to the uniqueness of each individual. Light touch will not reach the deepest of reflexes.

Another example: Based on traditional charts - has any of you ever worked on the neck area or the **pituitary** (pi-**two**-i-ter-ree) area of the great toe or the hip / sciatic and had the majority of clients express pain when those areas are worked? Almost all of my clients complain of discomfort and show marked sensitivity. Does that mean that every single one of them has a problem with their neck, low back or pituitary gland?

Or how about when you struck a reflex in a zone and pain ensued from the pressure, yet the client had no issues in any part of the zone? What about the individuals who had no pain in their feet as you made several passes over the entire foot, then after hitting a real zinger, the whole foot becomes sensitive?

Example: Let's say I started my reflexology treatment by immediately working the knee reflex or the transverse colon or the lungs. I would find that the vast majority of my clients would exhibit little-to-no pain even though I used intense pressure (excluding plantar fasciitis clients).

Now remember I'm working over those reflex areas and there is no sensitivity which usually means it's okay, right? Then I go to the amygdala reflex, strike it with minimal pressure and watch the client reel back in his chair in agony, yelling, *"What the heck was that?!"* Note that I used minimal pressure to receive that alarming response.

However, what is more interesting is I will go right back to those same reflexes I mentioned earlier and using LESS pressure than I did originally, the client would be jerking his feet; trying to get away from the pain. Now we have a reply of 'yes' from the brain.

It was this inconsistency that made me wonder: Why was an area that was insensitive all of a sudden sensitive and then after several passes became insensitive again? In performing treatments on many people over the years I noticed that my clients shared a commonality of the most sensitive (or dominant) reflexes. I also took note of how after working those more sensitive reflexes, the more minor reflexes would, in effect, 'open up' and become more sensitive to the client. It was as if they were given permission to join the conversation by tying into the party line. When this connection happens from unlocking the hierarchical reflexes the client will get what I call 'the buzz' (glowing,

Chapter 2 – What is Reflexology?

heavy eyes with a look of deep relaxation).

A new contradiction in pain?

The problem I started to see was this; is pain coming from the opening of the dominant reflex or is the pain from an issue in the referral area? Turns out it was both. In order to get communication working well amongst all the members you first have to break the defensive stance of hierarchical reflexes. This in itself gets a pain reply from the brain! Then, it is the member itself that must be looked at more in depth by the brain. If further issues exist, more pain may be given as a return reply.

Note: To make it more confusing let me throw one more condition in here; real congestion in the feet. Calcium and uric acid are just a few elements that block nerve pulses. When we free up congestion in the literal feet, it too can bring on pain because nerves may have been dormant from a lack of good circulation and now are responding.

If you were to tie your upper leg with a tourniquet, blood would no longer circulate to the nerves. Then once loosed, blood would flow freely. But the pain is very intense as a recalculation of the nerves and brain resumes with the fresh flow of blood.

Hierarchical Pain leads to new understanding.

This is what caused me to challenge Zone Therapy. It became clear that there are certain reflexes that always seem hypersensitive in people and by unlocking them, opened up ways to reach 'intermedial' and 'elementary' reflexes. Thus, striking reflexes is not staged in five imaginary lines from the anterior to the posterior aspects of the plantar surface (according to zone therapy), rather an outward sweeping motion from the distal aspect of the Hallux (**hal**-uhx) to the subsequent descending vitals.

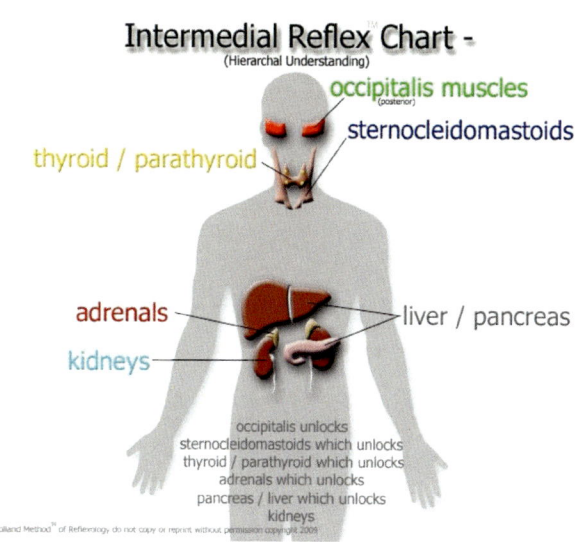

That's why even though you made passes earlier in the session and no pain occurred at certain reflex points, shortly, progressive new pains developed as exposure was now

18

Chapter 2 – What is Reflexology?

<u>available</u> from the opening of dominant reflexes.

If a massage therapist is to begin treatment with a client in the prone position, massaging glutes first and working his way down to the calves and then back up to the shoulders, would the client feel peak release and relief? No. Most therapists, in general, will tell you that people like to have their shoulders rubbed first, then their neck, followed by the rest.

The shoulders are worked first and then the neck because tension and stress is released systematically (hierarchal) in all humans. As a matter of fact, before you even touch a person, the atmosphere would be the most important beginning to a therapeutic treatment.

We all know what's best for us and what feels good and it's the same with the **dominant**, **intermedial** and **elementary** reflex system. They too are unlocked in a systematic, descending order.

Reflex chart on the following page.

Three Types of Reflexes		
Dominant	**Intermedial**	**Elementary**
This is the most important type of reflex. It requires less pressure to activate and open up sensitivity and communication to intermedial reflexes. This is the order I would recommend to work first.	*These are very important reflexes that, when struck, open and activate healing channels and communication to the elementary reflexes.*	*All other reflexes that help normalize the body. There is no particular order in how these reflexes influence each other.*
1) Amygdala / Brain (from brain to lower neck) – unlocks emotion and relieves all tension and stress due to anxiety. 2) Hypothalamus – unlocks parasympathetic and sympathetic systems. Controls the pituitary. 3) Pituitary / Pineal – unlocks chemical and hormonal systems and activates adrenals. Adjusts melatonin release. 4) Anterior / Posterior Trapezius (shoulders) – unlocks muscular system. 5) Sciatic / Hip / Pelvis – unlocks sciatic nerve and entire spine, and promotes circulation for the whole body. 6) Whole Spine – unlocks nerve supply to the entire body for internal diagnosis and healing.	1) Occipitalis – unlocks muscular tension in the back of neck unlocking the Sternocleidomastoid. 2) Sternocleidomastoid – unlocks tension in the neck and opens circulation to brain and thyroid. 3) Thyroid / Parathyroid – increase of energy by activating adrenals and decrease of overall inflammation. Adjusts calcium levels in blood. 4) Adrenals – unlocks fatigue due to stress and stimulates emotional well-being. 5) Liver – unlocks the cleansing abilities of the body. Detoxifies and aids the digestive system. 6) Pancreas – unlocks digestive system and regulates blood sugar. 7) Kidneys – unlocks chemistry of whole body functions and eliminates toxins.	- Sinus, Head, Eyes, Ears - Clavicles - Sternum - Heart, Pectoralis Major, Ribs, Esophagus, Bronchial, Breasts - Deltoids - Stomach - Gall bladder - Spleen - Arms, Hands, Elbows, Wrist, Biceps, Triceps - Colon, Small Intestines, Bladder, Ureters, Testes, Ovaries, Uterus, Prostate - Ileocecal Valve, Appendix - Legs, Knees, Achilles Tendons, Gastrocnemius, Hamstrings, Quadriceps - Latissimus Dorsi - Gluteus Maximus, Low Back

Chapter 2 – What is Reflexology?

What systems are involved with communication?

Congestion may be the link to bodily sickness. Think of communication between elements of the body in the same regard as communication between cities. In many ways one city can communicate with another. One way is by mail. Mail is physically brought from one city to another in a car or train. Another would be by flight or by phone and in more recent times digital signals such as TV or radio. The latest mode is the Internet.

Notice all these different ways of communication that have been recently invented or discovered. Now imagine that there are roadblocks on the roads due to roadwork, flights canceled because of weather, digital signal loss due to power outage and Internet service disrupted due to downed phone, cell or cable lines.

Organs, glands and parts of the body communicate with one another in both scientifically proven and unknown ways. The two most important means a reflexologist should note the communication are:

- The **Nervous System** - nerves transmit electrochemical messages to one another.
- The **Endocrine System** - endocrine glands communicate and regulate the body hormonally (chemically) and receive their instruction from the hypothalamus.

Powerful tools for opening communication.

The **Amygdala** (uh-**mig**-duh-luh) - the amygdala sends impulses to the **hypothalamus** (hy-puh-**thal**-uh-mus) for important activation of the sympathetic nervous system, handles emotional trauma and stress, as well as expressions of fear. Another task is for activation of dopamine, norepinephrine, epinephrine and serotonin. *In my opinion the amygdala is the most dominant reflex of the entire human system because it will dominate all systems of the body if it so chooses.*

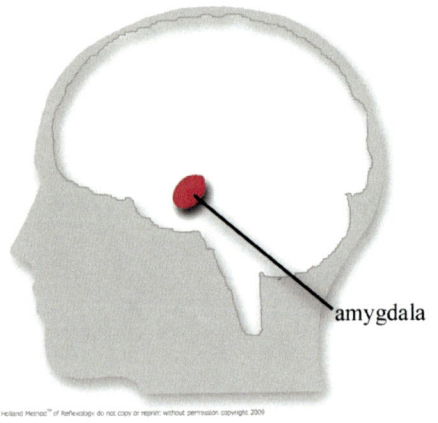

The hypothalamus connects two of the important communication systems. It is a tiny collection of nuclei that is responsible for controlling an infinite amount of behavior. I believe that reflexology is a genius at playing the subsystems of the **autonomic nervous system** (sympathetic nervous system / parasympathetic nervous system) against each other during the reflexology treatment. The amygdala spurs on this relationship and manifests itself as the controller of our emotional center. The hypothalamus also controls the thyroid.

The **sympathetic system** controls the body's response to emergencies. Known as the fight-or-flight response, this system responds by preparing your body to either fight the danger or flee. If a person breaks into your house and points a gun to your head, you would discover this system very quickly. This system raises blood pressure, heart rate, sweating and puts energy into the muscles.

The **parasympathetic nervous system** functions to counter the sympathetic system so that you don't make a serious mistake that could injure others or allow adrenalin to be released to the point that you blow a heart valve. After a crisis has passed, this system helps to calm the body. Heart and breathing rates slow, digestion resumes, pupil contraction and sweating cease.

Again, reflexes prod the brain to find and expose the blockage that hinders communication between body members and help it to decide if it needs to assist from within. <u>Pain is a result of the brain accepting this find</u>.

Members will defend themselves rendering true issues as forgotten.

We also have the example of masked pain via the body's response to defend itself. How can an organ, gland or part of the body get to the point where it no longer communicates pain and an individual becomes disconnected from the natural indications of trouble in the body? I came up with this illustration years ago to help explain that this process does exist.

<u>The rock in the shoe:</u>

If I put a rock in your shoe, initially it would be very painful. Over a period of time if the rock is not removed, your central nervous system makes a decision: Most likely your brain would ignore the pain by masking it so that you can go on and live a functional life. Within a short period of time you would no longer feel the rock in your shoe. What does that mean? Well, the body has learned to defend itself. You have to go on with life.

However, the problem still exists. The rock is still in the shoe. The body does not just compensate mentally. It must physically compensate for the abnormality thrust upon itself. The affected foot would change the walking gait of the individual. The hips would adjust for skeletal discrepancies. The spine will try to keep the vertical pendulum upright. The head will balance on an uneven spinal disposition. Now the whole body would have gone out of alignment (or out of homeostasis) because you're not walking properly.

So one day you decide that you're tired of the dysfunctional attitude of your body and now, with accruing pain manifesting itself in age, you – lo and behold – remove the rock in the shoe. You have now successfully removed the blockage causing disharmony of the entire center mass. The removal of the blockage causes new-found pain similar to the unblocking of a nerve impulse through the acupressure of reflexology. Both illustrate physical approaches (rock removed and reflex pressure) and able to expose the original corruption of the once balanced system and help the body to again normalize.

Now, is it conceivable that your body will return to the health and well-being in an instant, as if you removed the rock the day it was deposited in your shoe? Of course not. You now must re-establish the healing process in descending order, which takes time. This is what you would expect since what occurred in the body after the introduction of the rock was also a process in getting sick, and not an immediate reaction throughout the body.

The striking of reflexes achieves the same goal as removing the rock in the shoe. Remember, a reflex is the discovery of congestion by the brain with the aid of reflex pressure on the part of the practitioner. The rock needs to be removed so that the body can normalize and return to homeostasis (normal health). Once again, the channels of communication are restored between the body members (or the cities like in the illustration) via this unblocking process.

To diagnose or not to diagnose?

"My clients want me to diagnose, and you said not to, but are you sure you cannot pinpoint a health issue?"

Again, reflexes do not necessarily mirror or demonstrate a specific problem with an organ, gland or part of the body. A reflex response is the internal diagnosis by the brain, then subsequently, the unblocking of congestion that is found in, around, up to or between vitals.

We use the anatomical chart only to help the client see where the congestion lies in the

Chapter 2 – What is Reflexology?

body. *Reflexologists should not assume or convey to clients that this reflex demonstrates a marked problem with the human structure even though this might clearly be the case.*

To illustrate: Let's say I happen to be applying pressure in the adrenal reflex area. Pain ensues. The client says, "what is that on the chart?" I respond with, "adrenal reflex," with no explanation. I've just now implied the client has a problem with their adrenal glands. Even if this may be so, there is no possible way a reflexologist could dogmatically nor diagnostically make such a claim. Why? Think of how the endocrine system works. Who is the master of the adrenal glands? The thyroid. Who is the master of the thyroid? The pituitary (the master gland). What organ instructs the endocrine system through the pituitary? The hypothalamus.

So we find discrepancies in and around the adrenal area. Who's to blame? The client reports low energy after I've revealed the issue, confirming in his mind, 'this must be the case'. But as stated above it could be any of the other members responsible for the reported lethargy on the part of the client. How about the fact the client may have an extremely poor diet or a sedentary lifestyle? Do you see now why we need to, as professional reflexologists, address the entire physiological system and <u>not treat for a specific disease</u>?

Another example would be pain in the shoulder. An individual may assume that the pain in the shoulder or limitations placed thereof is a direct cause of their pain. I would argue that congestion leading up to the shoulder limits communication necessary for healing, circulation or correct nerve response. Once congestion is removed by reflexology stimulation, false pains may be discredited and disseminated by the brain as well as other active vitals. Think of this: when a pregnant woman experiences Braxton-Hicks (or false labor) contractions, is she in labor?

Three types of congestion I focus on:

1) Toxins that interfere with the biochemistry of the endocrine / lymphatic / digestive / nervous systems.
2) Improper defense and self-isolation of a vital member.
3) Loss of communication because of closed doors in hierarchal members.

There is no doubt that congestion exists on other molecular levels. However, as specialists in our field we give precedence to the main culprits of poor homeostasis.

Chapter 2 – What is Reflexology?

So why communicate anything to the client?

It is also the responsibility of the reflexologist to know how the anatomy and physiology of the body works. This knowledge is not to diagnose, but to get a better hold on the science and to alleviate concerns as well as preconceived notions of the client.

There are some really bad reflexologists out there, who make a mess of our modality – by making absurd claims and other falsehoods. We need to be prepared to make a defense when they become our client.

Even though you do not profess to be his doctor, some may view you as such. So it is our responsibility as reflexologists to explain what role we play in his overall health.

It is important to emphasize that his doctor (General Practitioner) is the one who is most responsible for his overall health care (after himself, of course). We are just a slice of the health care pie.

I believe there are six priority steps to achieve health. Over the years these steps have become quite clear and my clients have verbally confirmed my thinking with this hypothesis:

1. Emotional State
2. Rest
3. Diet
4. Exercise
5. Holistic Therapy
6. Physician

Holistic Therapy - of which Reflexology is a part - is a slice of the health care pie

Why is reflexology not the Number-One priority?

A good explanation to clients is this:

1) Reflexology is not a cure-all.
2) Reflexologists cannot prescribe medicine.
3) If a person is missing a limb, all the reflexology treatments in the world will not make it grow back.
4) Reflexology is to be viewed as preventive. If a person eats junk food all day,

reflexology will have little impact on their health.

Is it palliative? Individual clients of mine have viewed it to be so but caution is needed here. Example: One of my clients had severe diabetes and he claimed that my reflexology treatments helped lower and stabilize his blood sugar. This was a man who was careful with his health (did not suffer overweight and was under the care of his physician). I, of course, believed him but would the reflexology treatments have helped him if he ate candy bars all day, refused to exercise and see his doctor? Absolutely not. See points # 1 and #3. Reflexology is not a cure-all and in the case of this client, a Type I diabetic, his pancreas will probably not produce insulin ever again.

Another successful example I had been privileged to witness was the healing of my own health problem. My hands and feet sweated profusely throughout my teen years and early adult life. I was very difficult to handle a piece of paper because my hand got stuck to it. Changing socks two times a day was no fun either. Unable to find the cause of this problem through allopathic and holistic measures, I accepted the fact that I would have to deal with it for the rest of my life.

After many years of embarrassment, a new acquaintance expounded on how great he felt from a reflexology session. Curious as to what reflexology was, my initial optimism quickly turned to skepticism. It seemed ridiculous that someone would press spots on the feet and things would happen in other parts of the body. However, my feet did hurt most of the time, so if I gave the dude a try, he might at least help that issue, right?

Little did I know that Harold Charleston, who has been practicing reflexology for more than 30 years, would change my life forever. The session was very painful. If it was not for my pride as a man I would have run out the door as the first spike of pain ensued. It was as if pieces of glass and edges of metal nails were being driven into my flesh. My feet perspired at an insane rate, so much so, that Harold had to keep wiping my foot with a towel just to remain sanitary.

It was a beautiful sunny day as I headed back to my car. I felt drugged, tired and relaxed all at the same time and found it quite difficult to find my car which was parked just a few feet in front of me. The drive home was difficult due to my lethargy, and I could not wait to go to bed. I slept thirty-six straight hours, waking only to eliminate fluids from time to time. Once I awakened from hibernation the feeling of euphoria dominated. I quickly discerned my problem of inadvertent sweating was gone.

"How is that possible?" I thought. He acted as if this was the norm when he addressed the imbalance was in my endocrine system.

This started me on the path of researching holistic health and my journey to learn and practice reflexology. Join me on my path and then create your own.

Chapter 2 – What is Reflexology?

Chapter Three

The Anatomy of the Feet

Chapter 3 – The Anatomy of the Feet

Anatomy of the Feet

Foot Basics

I still seem to be amazed at the mechanical complexity and structural strength of the human foot. The daily punishment that people put their feet through should make them look like a bowl of chicken-chow-mein with a side order of rice pudding. Yet, the feet remarkably adapt to their environment allowing us to continue our life's course.

The bones of the feet act like shock absorbers, containing foundational strength, and withstanding thrust pressures that bewilder the mind. I have seen a teenager jump out of a tree approximately twelve feet high, landing on his bare feet and then walk away with a smile.

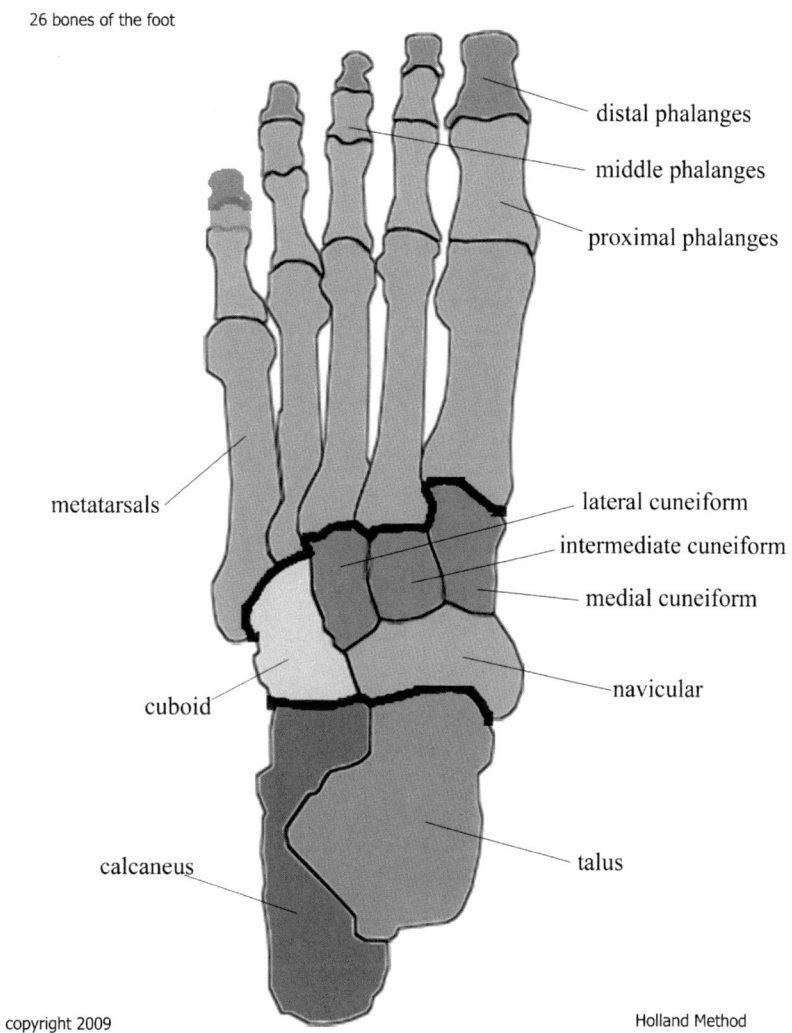

The entire foot assembly is comprised of 26 bones, 33 joints and more than 100 tendons, muscles, ligaments, and a membrane called fascia (**fash**-ee-uh) that connects these bones together. The bones can slightly articulate from one another because they are held together by these members.

I have noticed that when someone does not take care of his feet, uric acid is able to creep into the joints, as well as other elements - such as calcium, that are there trying to neutralize this acid - the bones will try to self-cast and bond, contributing to a loss of mobility, articulation and strength. Stretching and opening these structures help us maintain good circulation and mobility in order to reach the reflexes.

So what is that sound that is heard when the joints open from time to time? Gases build up in the synovial (si-**nov**-vee-el) fluid, and when gently opened they can release this build up of gas. Nitrogen is one of the suspected culprits. But don't worry, the fluid returns quickly and the gases will re-establish themselves within twenty to thirty minutes.

Let's Look at the Bones

I'll start with the most distal aspect of the foot: the **phalanges**. There are 14 **phalanx** (**fay**-lank-x) bones that play an important part of balance and propulsion. The hallux (or the big toe) has two bones (phalanxes) whereas digits 2-5 have three each.

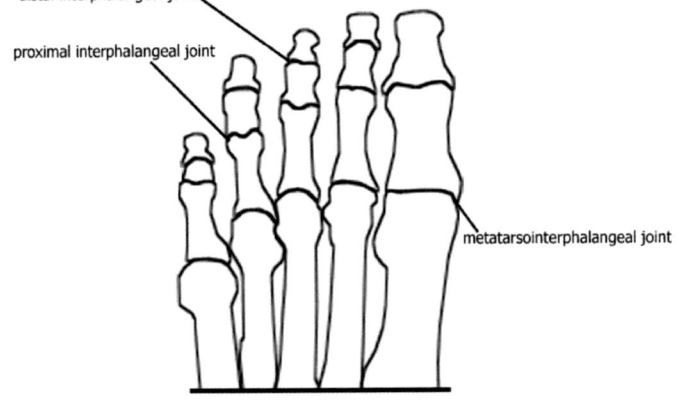

The joint that resides between the phalanxes is known as the **interphalangeal joint**. When referring to digits two through five we must distinguish which joint we are talking about.

- The **metatarsophalangeal joint** is where the metatarsal bones head meets the base of the phalanx.
- The **proximal interphalangeal joint** is where the head of the fist phalanx meets the base of the second.
- The **distal interphalangeal joint** is where the middle phalanx head meets the base of the last phalanx.

We only use the term interphalangeal joint when referring to the joint between the phalanges in the hallux because there are only two bones. It is very important to stretch, in an extension movement, these phalanges so that all the joints remains mobile allowing your fingers to penetrate deep to find those low-lying reflexes. I like to rotate the hallux many times during a session so that the articulation (ar-**tic**-you-**lay**-shun) of the head of the metatarsal's metatarsophalangeal joint remains sound.

There are 5 metatarsal (met-uh-**tar**-suhl) bones that join both the phalanges at the distal aspect and the 7 major bones at the proximal aspect (tarsals - / **tar**-suhl). We call this the midsection of the foot, and this is where your arch resides.

The 7 major bones of the foot and ankle are:
- **Talus** – (**tay**-less) the top of the talus is connected to the two long bones of the lower leg which is the tibia and fibula.
- **Calcaneus** – (kal-**kay**-nee-us) or better known as the heel bone. It is the largest bone in the foot.
- **Navicular** – (nuh-**vik**-you-ler) is the keystone of the medial arch.
- **Cuneiforms** (3) – (**kyoo**-nee-uh-form) the intermediate cuneiform is the keystone of the transverse arch lying between the lateral and medial cuneiforms.
- **Cuboid** – (**kyoo**-boid) this bone resides where a notch on the lateral aspect of the foot can be seen, making it easy to find. The cuboid is the keystone of the lateral longitudinal arch.

There are 3 arches in which the reflexologist should focus on: The **Medial Longitudinal Arch**, the **Lateral Longitudinal Arch** and the **Transverse Arch**.

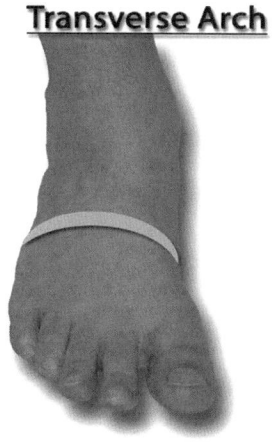

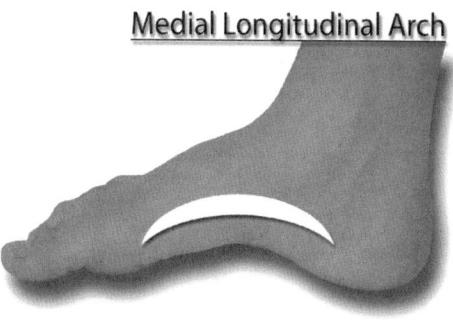

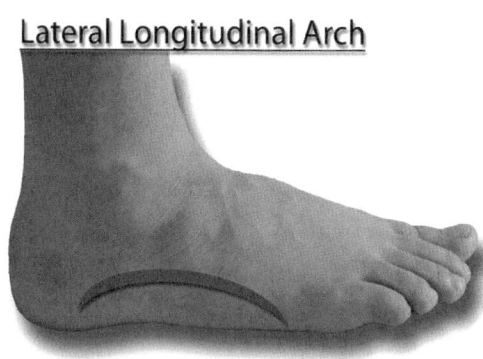

These 3 arches create the foundation of our health. If these arches are compromised in any way we will see the general performance of the body decrease. The medial longitudinal arch seems to receive the greatest of attention in the sports world because, as we know, this arch can make or break the athlete's speed and agility.

Chapter 3 – The Anatomy of the Feet

It has, however, gained the attention of multi-million dollar corporations interested in capitalizing on the public's diagnosis du jour - that everyone who has pain in the foot must have a problem with his medial arch. Thus we are bombarded daily with orthotics advertising.

In my opinion, this has been over-prescribed for the vast amount of people who complain of foot pain. In some cases, a client will tell me that he has thrown away his orthotics after receiving just a few reflexology sessions. *And here is why:* The entire anatomy of the foot works in harmony to absorb shock. This is of great importance to the spine for it too was designed to carry loads and handle bounce as well. If the spring of the medial arch is lost then the spine must carry this full responsibility on its own.

Unless a person is born deformed, the natural arch of a person should be nurtured holistically. Why? Because the mold (orthotic) now acts as a rigid, compressive structure that removes the 'spring' that needs to be there. With good circulation and mobility, the foot should bounce resulting in better overall health. However, there may be good reasons for helping the arch with supports if the person has severe pronation.

Pronation

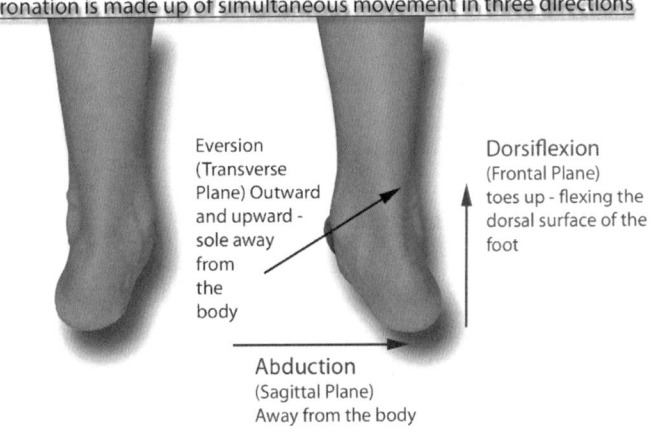

Pronation of the Foot

Pronation is made up of simultaneous movement in three directions

Eversion (Transverse Plane) Outward and upward - sole away from the body

Dorsiflexion (Frontal Plane) toes up - flexing the dorsal surface of the foot

Abduction (Sagittal Plane) Away from the body

The pronated foot is one in which the heel bone angles inward (medially) and the arch tends to collapse. This person may be considered flat-footed but not all flat-footed individuals have a pronated stance. A "knock-kneed" person has overly pronated feet. This flattens the medial arch as the foot strikes the ground in order to absorb shock when the heel hits the ground. The condition can become so severe that it appears the individual is walking on his talus bone.

When a client comes into your office with this issue and complains of ankle pain, it would be prudent to recommend a podiatrist or orthopedist to correct the condition. You may assist the primary physician by keeping circulation in the foot before and after surgery (if it is needed). As far as reflexology is concerned, this person could definitely benefit from relief due to the imbalances in his entire system.

Supination

Supination (soo-puh-**nay**-shun) in the foot occurs when a person appears "bow-legged" with their weight supported primarily on the lateral/anterior aspect of their feet. The more severe the supination of the foot, the more likely the ankle could roll completely over - tearing ligaments between the calcaneus and the talus bone. If someone has sprain / strained these lateral ligaments, be careful when applying medial flexion (adduction). If the injury is very acute, I would not even rotate the foot or articulate it in any direction during the session. Just stick to the **planar** reflexes. When the client's doctor gives you the 'all clear', then gently proceed.

Supination of the Foot

Supination is made up of simultaneous movement in three directions

Inversion (Transverse Plane) Inward and upward - sole toward the body

Plantarflexion (Frontal Plane) Toes down - flexing the plantar surface of the foot

Adduction (Sagittal Plane) Toward the body

Common Terms About the Arch:

- The term 'Flat-footed' applies to the arch which is sitting on the ground completely.
- Medium arches are sometimes called 'Normal arches'.
- Exaggerated arches are less common and referred to as a 'High arch'.

Muscles of the feet

We will not go over all the muscles of the foot, rather just focus on a few that should be of interest to the reflexologist. These two muscles, when torqued, free up the foot and provide room for increased circulation, which brings the **plantar** reflexes to the fore. **Dorsal** flexing and **lateral** flexing (abduction) of the foot should engage the muscles.

- The **Flexor digitorum brevis** lies in the middle of the sole of the foot, a muscle that flexes the second phalanx of each of the four small toes.
- The **Flexor hallucis brevis** lies in the anterior aspect of the foot and is divided into two portions, which are inserted into the medial and lateral sides of the base

of the great toe. The posterior position arises near the **medial** aspect of the cuboid bone.

Tendons of the Feet

Again, I will bring attention to just two tendons that reflexologists encounter daily.

- The **Flexor Hallicus Longus Tendon**, is a tendon that occupies nearly the whole length of the posterior surface of the flexor hallicus longus muscle and attaches at the base of the big toe. If you dorsal flex the Hallux, the tendon will protrude and become very sensitive to the reflexologist's touch. Be careful not to press too hard on this tendon. We would not want to hyper-extend the tendon, making the client sore for a few days. Gently stretch this tendon by following it from the posterior-medial position of the cuboid bone to the most distal aspect of the great toe.
- The **Achilles tendon**, also known as the **calcaneal tendon** is a tendon of the posterior leg. It serves to attach the **gastrocnemius** (calf muscle / gas-trok-**nee**-mee-us) muscle to the calcaneus (heel) bone. Working the posterior aspect of the heel will relax the gastrocnemius. That in turn will allow for greater range of motion for the foot and in particular, it's ability to dorsal flex.

Nerves of the Feet

Due to the complexity of the Nervous System and its periphery, there are too many nerves to enumerate but the most common estimate is 7,200.

Chapter 3 – The Anatomy of the Feet

Chapter Four

The Conditions That Can Affect the Feet

Conditions of the Feet

Arthritis

In recent years arthritis has increasingly plagued mankind and, in particular, citizens of the United States over the age of 50. Its many conditions have multiple faces with one goal in mind – to make your joints ache and hurt. The inflammation of the lining of the cartilage brings pain and discomfort, and in some cases, disability. My clients have revealed to me that they believe the root cause is from acid resulting from poor diet. We learn a lot from our clients and one example I would like to share with you deals with the disease of arthritis.

This particular client told me, "Doug, my doctor said uric acid enters the joint structure from the blood vessels. The acid comes in contact with my tissue and causes nerve receptors to call upon the brain to render aid. Aid comes in the form of calcium that is alkaline and will neutralize the offending acid." Well, he was right. One condition from uric acid that causes tremendous pain is Gout.

Gout

Excess uric acid crystals collect in and around the joints of the big toe. The Hallux's interphalangeal joint and metatarsointerphalangeal joint are commonly the focal point, due to the fact they remain the most distal aspect of the body. Being so far from the heart, circulation becomes the poorest – making a haven for crystals to collect easily – often leading to severe pain in the big toe.

Studies show that men are more likely to develop gout / arthritis than women. One of my male clients had it so bad that tears would be visible in his eyes with each step into my office. Since the gout was that acute, I suggested that he go to his physician and get medication to ease the pain and inflammation first. Working on acute gout could cause increased inflammation and be detrimental to the client's health. If the condition is not in its acute stage, by all means, let your light shine by bringing in good circulation to those distal extremities.

Osteo-arthritis

The most common type of arthritis is called osteoarthritis. Osteoarthritis causes loss of cartilage in the joints of the foot. Articulation of foot members becomes very difficult and painful. The pain and swelling worsens with each step or after periods of being off the feet for periods of time.

Be careful with stretching, rotating and the flexing of the clientss feet who has this condition. Most likely they are mature in age (above 70-years-old) and soundness of mind should be applied as to pressure, stretching and articulation any ways. Just remember, it took 70 years to get where he is at, let's not try to go for miracles in just a few visits.

Rheumatoid Arthritis

Another type of arthritis is rheumatoid arthritis and is known for being the most crippling form of the disease. It can cause severe deformities of the joints making it difficult to live a normal life. People who suffer from rheumatoid arthritis often develop severe forefoot problems such as bunions, hammer toes, claw toes, and other deformations of the toes. It is also known as an autoimmune disease that causes chronic inflammation of the joints.

Tarsal Tunnel Syndrome

Posterior Tibial Neuralgia (also known as Tarsal Tunnel Syndrome) is pain in the foot, ankle and toes caused by compression of or injury to the nerve supplying the heel (posterior tibial nerve).

The posterior tibial nerve clings to the back of the calf, through a fibrous canal (the tarsal tunnel) near the calcaneus, and into the plantar pad of the foot. Inflamed tissues around this nerve can then press on the nerve, causing discomfort. Some of the conditions that can cause tarsal tunnel syndrome would include edema, fracture, arthritis and gout which contribute to the inflammation of the joints.

The discomfort felt by my clients include: burning in and around the ankle, big toe and the back of the calf (gastrocnemius). Also, they describe intermittent tingling in the toes when sitting down or shooting pains from the back of the heel.

Make sure to work the hip / sciatic reflexes thoroughly in order to increase circulation and flexibility to the tarsal - fibula conjunction. Our goal is to assist the body in sending nutrients and blood flow to the tarsal tunnel fibers and its subsequent nerves for client health. It has been my experience that clients who have poor dorsal flexion exhibit these signs. Some have gone to their doctor and received corticosteroid shots to relieve inflammation. By working the hip / sciatic reflexes as well as the gastrocnemius reflexes, we assist the doctor to achieve the doctor / patient goals.

Calluses

Believe it or not, calluses are a good thing even though they may hurt occasionally. Calluses show up where friction exists on the skin. If it was not for the body forming a callus on an area receiving friction, the skin would open up a major wound and that would allow for the severing of blood vessels and, possibly, infection and death.

The body uses dead skin cells that harden over the area of the foot where the friction occurs. You will see calluses just about anywhere on the foot but primarily on the heel, hallux, smallest toe or on the heads of metatarsals two and three. Again, improper shoes cause the majority of foot problems, calluses in particular.

Make sure to work the reflexes right over the top of these calluses. Do not baby the calluses. We want to increase circulation in and around the affected area. If the calluses are infected refer them to their doctor immediately.

Corns

Corns are very similar to calluses in the sense that they are formed from an accumulation of dead skin cells on the foot creating hardened areas. The difference is that they contain a cone-shaped core with a point that is notorious for finding and pressing on a sensitive nerve below, causing unusual pain. One client told me "Doug, it's like stepping on a nail all day long." Corns become inflamed for the same reason that calluses form: friction. With regards to how corns actually develop, refer to 'Calluses' above.

Diabetes and the Foot

Diabetes affects approximately 20 million Americans and is categorized into two different types: Type I and Type II.

- Type I is usually hereditary and is also referred to as Juvenile Diabetes because its onset is usually in childhood.
- Type II, also referred to as Adult Onset Diabetes and (even though it can be hereditary) it is usually the result of poor diet.

Here's how Type II diabetes presents: Let's say a person eats a large amount of sugar and simple carbohydrates throughout the years. The pancreas, which produces insulin (that utilizes the sugars for energy), becomes worn out. Low blood sugar occurs as the pancreas gets used to flooding the blood with insulin to break down these sugars. So blood sugar levels are regularly unstable.

After years of pancreatic abuse, the pancreas can no longer keep up with the demand to produce insulin at such high levels. As the pancreas begins to under-perform, everyday functions start to suffer. Without insulin, the food we eat is not processed adequately for energy and then blood sugar levels start to rise. Diabetes (high blood sugar) disrupts the vascular system by attacking the kidneys, eyes, legs and feet.

It has been estimated that 25% of all American diabetics will develop foot-related problems. We are going to pay particular attention as to how diabetes affects circulation and neuropathy.

Neuropathy

Diabetic Neuropathy causes numbness in the feet. My clients tell me that you lose the ability to feel pain, heat or cold. They may even become unaware of cuts or bruises on their toes or feet due to the loss of sensitivity. For instance, I was working on this client recently; after inspecting the feet, as I always do before I start the session, I noticed her fourth digit on the right foot was significantly bruised. I asked her, "Did you drop something on your toe or stub your foot?" Her reply was, "I didn't even know I had injured it. I feel no pain there."

This is why it's very important to inspect the feet before each treatment, especially in the case of those with Diabetic Neuropathy. If you discover a cut or infection on a Type II

Diabetic, inform them to go to their doctor immediately. Due to poor circulation and high sugar levels in the blood, infection can easily set in and the client can actually lose digits or limbs.

Poor Circulation

Peripheral Vascular Disease is often caused by diabetes, which hinders the circulation of blood down the legs to the feet. The reduced oxygen and nutrition needed for healthy feet cause a host of issues: swelling, dry skin, toe fungus, hard nails, poor healing, loss of sensation, poor balance, loss of dorsal flexion, stiff toes, plantar fasciitis, etc.

When working on a diabetic it may take several passes over the planar surface to stimulate localized nerves in the dermis, at which, the client will get a rush of pain or other strange sensations that they have not felt for some time because of the lack of blood flow to the nerves.

Nerves need blood to give proper feedback and contribute to internal diagnoses for the needs of the feet and other extremities. When blood is cut off due to poor circulation those responsibilities are hindered and thus we see the foot problems that we do. We're going ahead of ourselves right now but not only would I work the pancreas reflex area but I would try to stimulate the kidneys, the whole spine and the low back to bring relief to the client.

Some people do not want to make the necessary dietary changes to alleviate the symptoms of their diabetes (which, in my opinion, is the first thing they SHOULD do) so stay off that soapbox and bring them as much relief as possible through reflexology.

Plantar Fasciitis

Plantar fasciitis (**plan**-tar **fash**-ee-**eye**-tis) is a painful inflammatory condition of the arch of the foot caused by excessive wear or stretching of the plantar fascia. My clients tell me that the first few steps of their day is like stepping on hot pokers or broken glass. They try to grab walls, dressers or loved ones in order to stay upright until the pain subsides. It is a heck of a way to start your day. The reason they feel pain is because while they were resting, the plantar fascia contracted back to its original shape. So during the first few steps of the morning the foot bones try to stretch the arch fascia to give the foot bounce and prepare it to handle load.

Being overweight has been one of the leading contributors to Plantar Fasciitis. Obesity, weight gain, jobs that require a lot of standing or walking on hard surfaces such as concrete, as well as women who wear high heels because 'the current mode of fashion dictates it', do a great disservice to the feet, which contribute to this condition. But we have to work on our feet, and there is no getting around that.
Dealing with hard surfaces is just a part of life.

Plantar fasciitis often results in a heel spur on the calcaneus (anterior), in which case it is the underlying condition, and not the spur itself, which produces the pain. The reflexologist can feel the spur if it is large enough. It has been my experience that while striking reflexes in the area of the plantar surface, the symptoms of plantar fasciitis is relieved. No doubt, fresh blood is introduced as toxins are flushed out of the fascia area causing the membrane to become more fluid in nature.

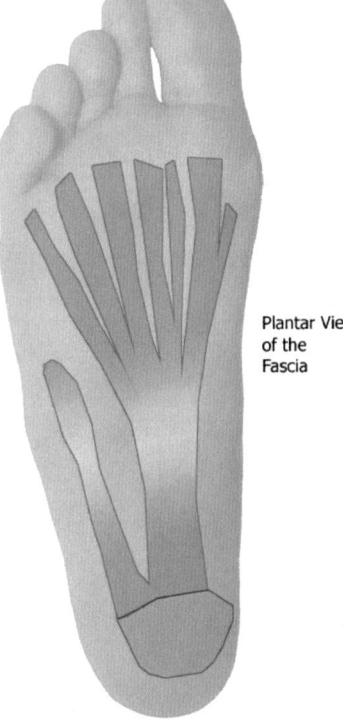

Plantar View of the Fascia

Remember to work the plantar surface carefully so as not to give the client too much pain. The condition did not start overnight and giving assistance through the striking of reflexes will take time also.

What is Plantar Fascia?

A ribbon-like membrane expansion or connective tissue, serving mainly to connect a muscle with the parts that it moves. Think of thousands of strands of tendon-like materials, interwoven for strength, yet flexible enough for the foot to articulate in many directions.

Heel Spur

A heel spur is a bony protrusion that hooks out of the bone and is associated with plantar fasciitis. This calcium formation is born from friction and stress to the fascia and to the bone.

The bone that seems to be the most affected is the calcaneus, especially on the anterior aspect of the plantar surface. This is where the plantar fascia meets the calcaneus bone. It is also where the most amount of pressure and strain from physical use is concentrated. 'Heel Spurs' can be seen by x-ray and is a term easier to express than 'plantar fasciitis'.

It has been reported that roughly 75% of persons with plantar fasciitis have a heel spur that can be seen by x-ray. In some instances, we can also feel them by palpating the soft tissue of the foot in and around the calcaneous during the reflexology session.

Make sure that you work directly on the spur with the permission of the client, because it may be painful to the touch. Work the tissue in all directions on and around the spur using strong acupressure. I have found that many times the spur dislodges on its own and the inflammation goes away.

Even though we do not treat for this specific condition, this positive response has been a pleasant surprise benefit for the client and practitioner. If the problem remains acute for the client, refer them to a podiatrist for further assistance.

Metatarsalgia (met-uh-tar-**sal**-gi-uh)

When the heads of the middle metatarsals (second, third and fourth) are crushed or cramped for space they will either rise in the center, or dip below the transverse arch line to avoid compression. This condition is called Metatarsalgia. Some women will beg their husbands to rub the ball of their foot because the pain from tissue inflammation between the metatarsals can be intense. Imagine wearing shoes all day long that bang your bones together from the outer sides.

This condition, when left untreated, can result in a sister condition called **Morton's Neuroma.** The most common location for a neuroma on the foot is between the third and fourth metatarsals and toes. This problem usually has symptoms that include a burning or tingling sensation from a swollen nerve in the ball of the foot that radiates out to the third and fourth toes.

Working on a foot with these conditions requires discernment. Rubbing the ball of the foot is one thing, driving your thumb between the metatarsal bones is another. Therefore, you must slowly work up through the webbing, providing fresh blood and circulation before the reflexes can really come to the fore. This will be very painful to the client.

Again, high-heeled shoes or improperly fitted shoes can be causal. Have I blamed shoes enough?

Achilles Tendonitis

The **Achilles tendon** is the large tendon located in the back of the leg that inserts into the heel, and can become inflamed due to degeneration or compression of the tendon. The only time this would be a concern to me would be if I was dorsal flexing or extending the foot. If someone tells you that they have this acute condition, just avoid stretching techniques until the problem subsides.

The most common cause is over-pronation of the foot which adds stress on the Achilles tendon. However, sudden sprinting and stopping of the legs during sports can also add to the problem. One of my clients slipped on ice to bring about an acute state of Achilles Tendonitis. Pay particular attention to the heel reflexes to bring relief to client under these circumstances.

Athlete's Foot

There are very few reasons why I would not work on a client's foot. Athlete's Foot is one of them. A reflexologist needs to learn to identify this condition quickly and how to handle the client's feelings tactfully.

Athlete's foot is a fungal infection that causes dry, red, flaking skin, sometimes accompanied by pain or itching. The feet will most likely smell. Look between the toes or on the soles or sides of the feet. In its acute stage, the infected foot exhibits blisters that weep and cause the client to itch. It can make its way to the dorsal aspect of the foot but this is rare.

Poor hygiene is the main culprit in getting this discomforting condition. In most cases the client has been in or around the pools and showers of a recreational center where mold spores thrive. Mold loves dark, moist places! And, because the fungi is present at the time the client steps barefoot on the surface of its dwelling, we see the fungi make its way to our office in the form of Athlete's foot..

Clients must keep their feet clean with soap and water and follow through with drying them thoroughly. Dry, clean feet as well as a healthy immune system repulse 'fungi squatters' allowing the client to receive the benefits from a reflexology session. In almost ten years of my practice, I have had only one client with this condition but unaware he had it. I believe anyone with an acute stage of Athlete's Foot would not schedule an appointment out of embarrassment anyway. So if this situation arises, tactfully educate them on what you think it may be, and ask if they have had the condition before. Let them know you cannot work on the feet as long as the condition is present for your and the rest of the clients' health and safety. Make sure you disinfect your chair as well as your hands, clothes, and carpet leading up to the chair.

Dry Skin

Most clients keep their feet clean. Dry skin is common even on clean feet. Don't be afraid to work on a foot that has dry skin. It won't hurt you. Just clean your floor of excess skin so as to remain sanitary for future clients.

Clubfoot

Clubfoot describes a range of congenital foot abnormalities in which the foot is twisted out of shape or position. The term "clubfoot", like a golf club, refers to the way the foot is positioned at a sharp angle to the ankle. It is a common birth defect and is usually an isolated problem for an otherwise healthy newborn although it can present with other birth defects, such as spina bifida. In most cases, clubfoot twists the top of the foot downward and inward, increasing the arch and turning the heel inward. The foot may be turned so severely that it actually looks as if it's upside-down.

However, because I do not work on young children, it is rare to come across this condition, except post-surgery. What you may notice in a clubfoot client is fused tarsal bones or lack of the ability of the foot to move adductionally.

****

You will become acquainted with many more conditions in addition these during your reflexology career. I hope this chapter helped you get an overview of what your responsibilities might entail.

Chapter Five

The Conditions of the Toes

Deformities or Conditions of the Toes

As a reflexologist you will come across certain toe deformities or conditions in your practice. I'll go over the most common ones I've contended with. But let me expound on my major pet peeve so that it's out of the way: Shoes, shoes, shoes. Did I mention shoes? I cannot stress enough how those in modern society voluntarily deform their toes by wearing improper shoes. Shoes take the lion's share of the blame, however, muscle imbalances and arthritis can also affect the feet.

The **hammer toe**, **claw toe**, and **mallet toe** are three separate conditions of the second, third, and fourth digits of the foot that have many similarities between them. They cause pain, inflammation and calluses. Each of the digits (excepting the hallux) has three bones. The deformities listed above are all due to abnormal positions of the bones at the joints between the bones.

Claw Toes

One question that I receive frequently from my older, female patients is, 'Can you straighten out my toes?' They are referring to their 'claw toe' or 'hammer toe'.

A claw toe is a toe that is contracted at the proximal or distal interphalangeal joints (middle and end joints in the toe), which presents itself as a cat's extended claw. When a muscle imbalance occurs, tendons and ligaments (plantar and collateral) cause the toe joints to curl downward. Arthritis, neuromuscular conditions or stroke can also contribute to the disorder. Clients will talk about pain on the tips of their toes because of the downward pressure from the condition. I've even seen some pretty nasty calluses on the ends of the toes because of this condition.

With claw toes the mobility of the toe joints are classified two ways: flexible and rigid. In a flexible claw toe, the joint has the ability to move. This type of claw toe can be manually straightened. I recommend reflexologists straighten and strike reflexes up or down the anterior position of the toes. This will not hurt the client and yet will bring great relief through stimulation of nerves in the area.

A rigid claw toe lacks that same ability to move due to the self-fusion of the interphalangeal joint. Movement is very limited and can be extremely painful. Extension movements should not be performed on rigid toes. Not only will this cause the client a great deal of pain but there is the small possibility of hyper-extending a ligament/tendon which would take several days for the soreness to dissipate. Gently rubbing the toes can bring needed circulation back into the region.

However, I do recommend that you work the posterior aspect of the digits the same way you would on a person that does not have this condition. Most likely this client will have calluses on the ends of their toes or at the peak of their phalangeal joints on the dorsal aspect. Work the toes regardless. Never try to remove calluses. That is what the podiatrist is for.

Mallet Toes

The mallet toe is the deformity where the most distal interphalangeal joint points downward and cannot straighten. This is most common in the second digit in persons whose second toe is the longest toe (or Morton's Toe) of the foot.

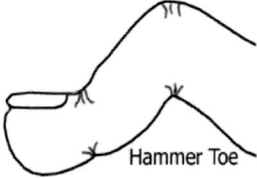
Mallet Toe

During your inspection of the feet at the beginning of the session, you will notice calluses on the forefront of these toes. They are quite painful for the sufferer but I recommend working them thoroughly, regardless of how thick the calluses are. Use sound judgment as to how much pain the client can tolerate to receive the future benefits. I always tell my clients: "You can either have a little pain with me voluntarily during this short session, or pain on a hospital gurney involuntarily – it's your choice?" That will get you a smile from time to time.

It is important to note that the plantar aspect of the interphalangeal joint will have a lighter appearance on the skin due to the constricted blood flow from the tightening of tendons / ligaments. Gentle extension of this toe is needed to bring blood back to the joint area and to the most distal region of the toe. This will stimulate the anterior trapezius reflexes in the upward motion.

Hammer Toes

A hammer toe occurs when the middle phalanx protrudes upwards, abnormally, at the proximal interphalangeal joint, like the dorsal fin of a shark. A painful callus often forms on the dorsal aspect of this joint from the toe rubbing against the shoe which could bring about a large amount of pressure and pain.

Ligaments and tendons that have tightened because of muscle imbalances or arthritis cause the toe's joints to curl downwards. As in mallet toes, the hallux is exempt from this condition.

Similar to the claw toe, the hammer toe needs to be extended manually for circulation and for the ability to reach reflexes. Remember the distinction of flexibility and rigidity in a claw toe? Likewise, follow the same formula in your approach to the hammer toe.

Morton's Toe

Morton's Toe is a disorder where the second digit is longer than the Hallux. The way the toes should be formed is that the hallux is the longest, followed by digits 2-5 in descending order. Unfortunately for those with Morton's Toe, their second digit is longer than their Hallux. This creates an oddity when wearing shoes and places greater pressure on the second digit because of its unnatural positioning.

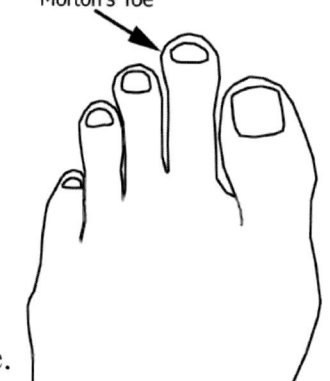

To clarify, imagine that while you are walking the foot balances itself by first engaging the most distal aspect of the hallux which bends first. This is followed by the second bone in the hallux. While the second bone engages, all other toes engage also and distribute pressure equally. This is not the case for a Morton's toe. The second digit engages the step first followed by the hallux and then the rest of the digits. It doesn't seem like it would be any big deal unless you have the problem. This is because the shoes, which are designed for normal feet, jam the cexond toe in so as to put the hallux in the first position. This can cause pain to the second toe as well as calluses and blisters.

Make sure to work the toe thoroughly through extension and rotation movements as well as up / down reflex driving of the anterior / posterior aspect of the toe to bring relief to the client.

Bunions

Hallux Valgus is a prominent bump on the medial side of the foot around the big toe's metatarsophalangeal joint. Clients are more familiar with the term 'bunions' and that is how they will refer to their condition when talking to you on the first reflexology session (the name 'hallux' refers to the big toe in the medical terminology).

The big red bulge on the side of the foot, as well as the large toe crossing other digits (overlapping toes), is hard to miss, and upon seeing this you would have instant compassion for the pain your new client is going through.

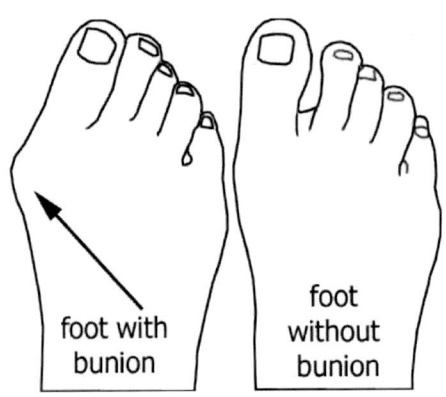

The reason they have this problem could be heredity, but I find it is more of a result of the client's history in not wearing proper shoes. Women in particular have destroyed their feet in the name of fashion. Tight pointy shoes and boots, or high-heels that push the phalanges into the bottom of a "snow cone" (so to speak), force and distress the natural foot structure to the point the toes no longer perform their function. By the time a person wakes up to the real reason behind this problem, it is usually too late. The foot is deformed. However, we can bring relief to the client by increasing circulation to the region through the articulating and stretching of the toes.

Another type of bunion which some individuals experience is called a Tailor's Bunion, also known as a 'bunionette'. I can never say that term correctly so I call it 'Baby-Bunion'. This forms on the lateral side of the foot at the 5th metatarsophalangeal joint (the little toe). It is a smaller bump that forms due to the little toe moving inwards, towards the big toe. Again, a result of the snow cone effect.

Pain comes from the inflammation, swelling, and soreness on the side surface of the hallux. The discomfort commonly causes a patient to walk improperly. I observed them decreasing their gait to avoid pressure on the distal aspect of the hallux and walking in a supine manner so that the lateral part of their foot, not the painful big toe, takes the brute force of daily walking. The best way to alleviate the pain associated with bunions is to wear proper fitting shoes.

Webbed Toes

Quite frankly, I am amazed how many clients have this condition also known as **syndactyly** of the feet. The condition presents itself as two or more digits of the feet fused together in a webbing of skin and flexible tissue. It has been so common to see this over the last ten years I began wondering if it was normal to have this condition; it is as normal as 'some people have blue eyes and some people have brown eyes'. Okay, I know that is an exaggeration, but – it is uncanny.

It's funny, I don't even notice it any more and yet the client will usually express a need for me to acknowledge what to them may be an embarrassment. After cordially doing so, I let them know that not only are they not alone, but it is more common than they would think.

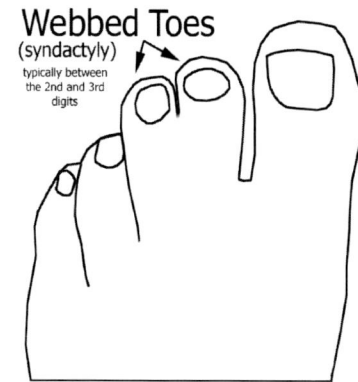

I wish I would have started a formal study and gathered hard data on just how many people I've seen with this condition. Just throwing out a number would be 1 out of 20 for the Northeast area of Ohio that I practice in. It is of interest to note that there are statistics that quote "1 out of 2,000 to 2,500 occurrences," with this condition, which has led me to believe either this data is completely wrong or that there is an unusual need for persons with webbed toes to see me for reflexology.

Toenail Fungus

Onychomycosis (**on**-i-koe-my-**koe**-sis) is one condition that you will definitely come across as a reflexologist. I have read surveys that say from anywhere up to 50% of Americans get fungus of the toenails by at least the age of 70. For whatever reason, the likelihood of getting it increases with age.

You will see the outward appearance of toenail fungus in many ways including: yellowing, thickening or crumbling of the nail, white streaks or stripes, spots, swelling or high arches in the nail. Sometimes the problem will be of such severity they will lose their nail entirely.

As a side note, a client of mine gave me a tip that worked well for him in getting rid of the toenail fungus. He used wild oregano oil in droplet form and put two drops three times daily directly on the nail itself. I was impressed at seeing his nails four or so months later looking pristine as if they belonged to a young teenager. He recommended the P73 oregano oil in extra virgin olive oil. Use your computer's search engine to find the different brands that carry this type of oregano oil.

Do not be afraid to work in and around the toes of a client with this condition. I have yet to hear of any reflexologist who has been adversely affected by doing so. I personally have never had any issue working with clients with toenail fungus. Just make sure to use an anti-bacterial agent on your hands before treating someone else (which you would do anyway no matter how good the condition of your client's foot). This, however, should not be confused with Athlete's Foot. That foot fungus is highly contagious and can spread quickly.

Diabetics have an increased risk of contracting onychomycosis because their immune system is compromised. It is my opinion the greatest contributor to toenail fungus is a compromised immune system which is spurred on by abnormal pH levels in the blood and in the skin. Look to acidosis as the primary culprit to fungus of any sort in the human system.

Ingrown Toenails

Onychocryptosis (ahn-i-**koe**-krip-**toe**-sis) simply means the condition of having an ingrown toenail. The nail grows into the nailbed causing pain and discomfort. The nail may even cause serious infection for those with weak immune systems, in particular Type 2 diabetics.

Remember I mentioned that there are only a few reasons why I wouldn't work on particular aspects of a foot? This would be another one of them. Do not work on the swollen skin of an acute ingrown toenail unless you want the client to kick you with his other foot. Why do people get ingrown toenails? Improper cutting or trimming of the nail or very tight shoes. *And I know this is common sense but for the uncommonly insensible* - never, ever, ever, ever, ever cut a client's toenails for them! If any infection ensues from your performing a service that you are not qualified to do, you will not 'pass go or collect $200'! Unless you are actually state-licensed, do not do it. I mention this because I have been asked many times by many of my clients if I can do this for them. It will come up for you, too.

****

This list is by no means exhaustive and reflexologists in different areas may see other conditions more common to them than these. More may be added in the future as the general state of people's health seems to worsen.

Chapter 5 – The Conditions of the Toes

Chapter Six

Understanding the Charts

Chapter 6 – Understanding the Charts

Understanding the Charts

Let us begin by familiarizing ourselves with the **foot chart** found at the end of this chapter. The purpose of the foot chart is to help you and the client get a general understanding of where the reflexes lie in the body and, eerily enough, how they correlate to the anatomical position.

We will include technical terms and it is best to learn these as it will actually make learning and performing reflexology easier. Terms like 'left', 'right', 'bottom' and 'top' become confusing depending on which direction you face. That's why sailors use positional terms like 'stern', 'aft', 'starboard' or 'bow' to pinpoint exact location no matter where they are stationed on a ship.

An important note: Something that confuses many students is, 'Why is medial and lateral on the hand different from medial and lateral on the feet?' Medial, as far as the anatomical position of the hands are concerned, is the outside of the hand. All medical charts demonstrate the human anatomy with the thumbs out and palms facing out.

Now imagine you're looking directly into the face of your best friend. Take the bottom of his two feet, make a copy of the bottom (or plantar surface) and visualize placing them close together and superimposing them over his body. So here's what it should look like: The two big toes should be covering the face. The two toes together represent the head. The little toes should cover the shoulders. The arms should run down the outer edge (or lateral side) of the feet. The spine runs down the very center of your friend's body to the groin. The heels should edge just past the thighs.

The left foot covers the left side of the body from the spine to the lateral aspect. The right foot covers the right side of the body from the spine to the lateral aspect.

Burn this image into your mind: That the feet together with the toes up are similar to the

Chapter 6 – Understanding the Charts

anatomical position (upright) of the human body, facing forward. If you stay with this thinking as you work the feet you will know pretty much where you are as regards to the anatomy and physiology of the human body.

Some general terms to know: If you stand up on your feet and look down at your feet, you are looking at the **dorsal** aspect of your feet. You are standing on the **plantar** surface of your feet. If there was ink on the ground and you stepped in it and walked across white paper, you would see the prints of your plantar surface. Still standing, try to put your feet together as tight as tight can be. Those two parts of your feet that have come in contact are the **medial** or inside of your feet. The **lateral** would then be the outside of your feet.

Standing up, standing on your head or sitting down or spinning around, these aspects of your feet never change. The dorsal is always the dorsal no matter how you're oriented.

If you were to stub your big toe, that would be the **distal** (or the furthest) aspect of your foot. The opposite would be the heel which is the **proximal** (or closer) part of your foot. The proximal aspect is the part of my heel that my kid hits when she insists on pushing the grocery cart behind me.

There are four guidelines that you need to become familiar with regarding the Holland Method reflexology chart:

- The Clavicle Guideline
- The Cuboid Oblique Guideline
- The Cuboid Transverse Guideline
- The Hip / Sciatic Guideline

These guidelines are designed to help us to see where we are in the feet with anatomical understanding.

The Clavicle Guideline is an imaginary horizontal line that separates the shoulders and head from the rest of the body. The reflexes that lie superior to the clavicle line are the trapezius, the neck, the sternocleidomastoid, the pineal / pituitary / hypothalamus, sinus / head / eyes / ears / thyroid / parathyroid, the cervicals and, finally, the brain / amygdala. This would also include all vital tissue, nerves, tongue, etc.

The Cuboid Oblique Guideline is an imaginary diagonal line that starts at the

Chapter 6 – Understanding the Charts

tuberosity of the fifth metatarsal base at the **cuboid notch** and goes to the base of the sternum. I created this diagonal line to split dead center of the liver in the right foot and the stomach and the pancreas of the left foot.

This makes it easy to separate the lung, kidney and adrenal of each foot. Obviously the lungs will be superior to the oblique guideline and the kidneys would be inferior.

I will give credit to my students if they include 'gallbladder' with the striking of the liver on the cuboid oblique guideline of the right foot. Subsequently I will give the same credit for student including the 'spleen' with the stomach reflex according to the cuboid oblique guideline of the left foot. The idea is that they are generally close to those vitals.

The reflexes that lie <u>superior to the oblique guideline</u> are the sternum, heart / pectoralis major / lungs / ribs / esophagus / bronchial / breasts, upper arm, upper thoracics of the spine and deltoid. The reflexes that lie <u>inferior to the oblique line</u> up to the transverse line are the adrenal glands / stomach / kidneys, liver /gallbladder (right foot), lower thoracics of the spine and the pancreas / spleen (left foot).

The Cuboid Transverse Guideline is an imaginary line running across the foot that separates the lower extremities from the transverse colon to the hip / sciatic guideline. Inferior to this guideline and superior to the hip sciatic guideline are the lumbar spine, colon / small intestine / bladder / ureters, ileocecal valve / appendix (left foot), testes / ovaries / uterus / prostate.

The Hip Sciatic Guideline is an imaginary line that separate the lowest region from the rest of the anatomical structure. It follows the change of skin (from soft to firm) at the plantar pad and has a mild transverse arch that follows the firm skin's line. The reflexes that are below this line are sacral-coccygeal, hip-sciatic / low back / pelvis, and then the legs / knees / achilles tendons / gastrocnemius / hamstrings / quadriceps.

By learning these terms, you could explain to a friend, by phone, two thousand miles away what you are talking about. For instance, if you look to the superior position of the clavicle you will notice there are many reflexes of interest. Let's describe the position of one of these reflexes in the right foot using these technical terms.

Put your finger on the inferior, lateral position of the hallux. What reflex is that? If you were not sure, I'd tell you to look above the Clavicle guideline. You would then notice that there are five toes and then you would try to discern what the name hallux means,

Chapter 6 – Understanding the Charts

which means 'big toe'. You would then ask yourself, 'What side of the big toe is the lateral side?' Facing the right foot, it would be the left side. Then you would try to discern what 'inferior' means, in other words – the lowest point. That would put you right at the beginning of the sternocleidomastoid (**stir**-know-**kly**-doe-mast-oid) from the lateral aspect.

Let's try another: What might be a reflex found in the inferior position of the cuboid oblique guideline near the most medial aspect of the left foot? It would lie superior to the right kidney and lateral of the spinal column. Have you figured it out yet?

Well, to be honest, <u>my chart does not show where the 'specific organs, glands and parts of the body lie perfectly' if at all</u>, so a general understanding of anatomy would tell you that a particular gland that is in a superior position to the kidneys and is lateral from the thoracic region would be *approximately* there. If you guessed the 'adrenal glands', you guessed correctly. However, if you guessed 'pancreas' you might still get credit for it.

Chapter 6 – Understanding the Charts

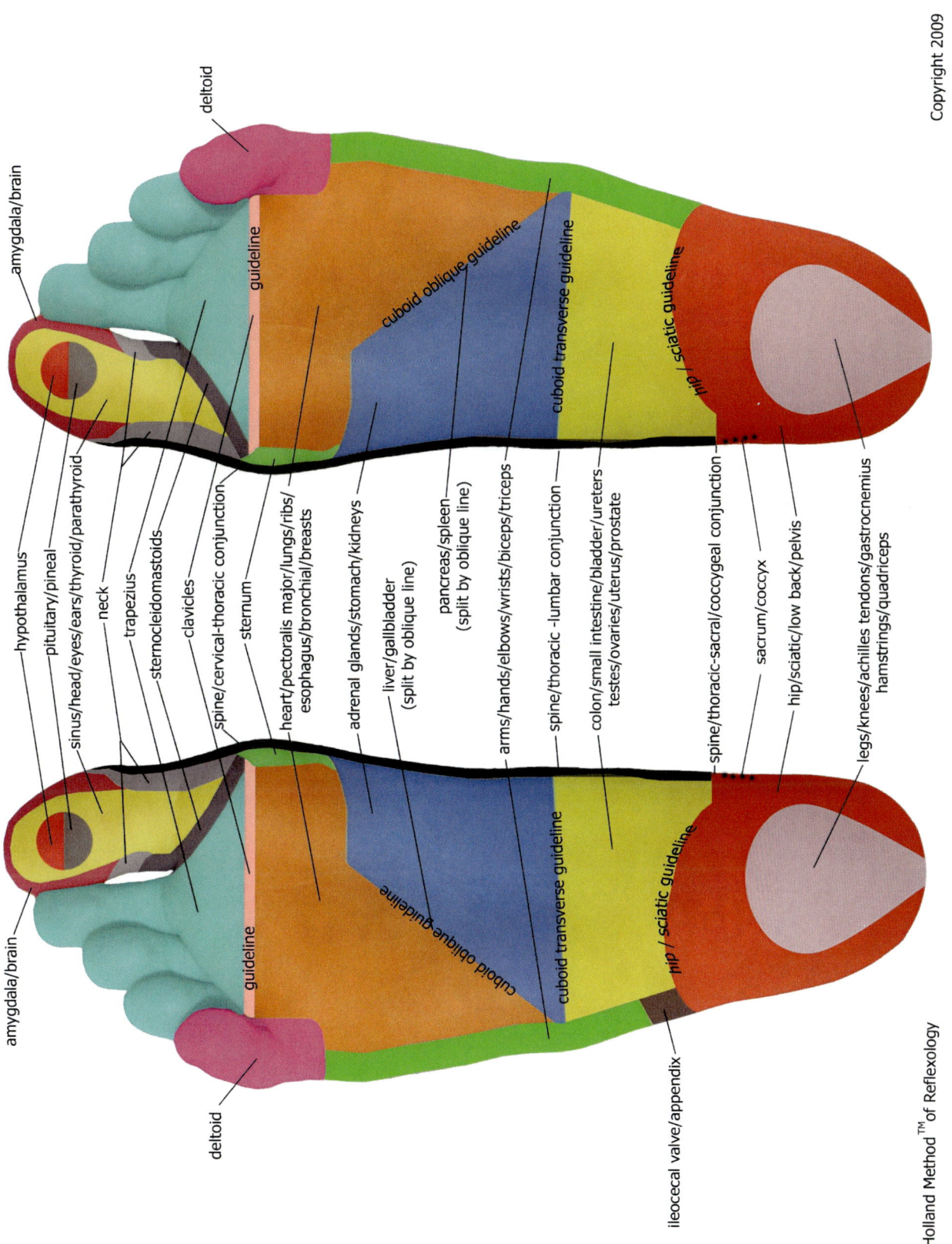

Chapter 6 – Understanding the Charts

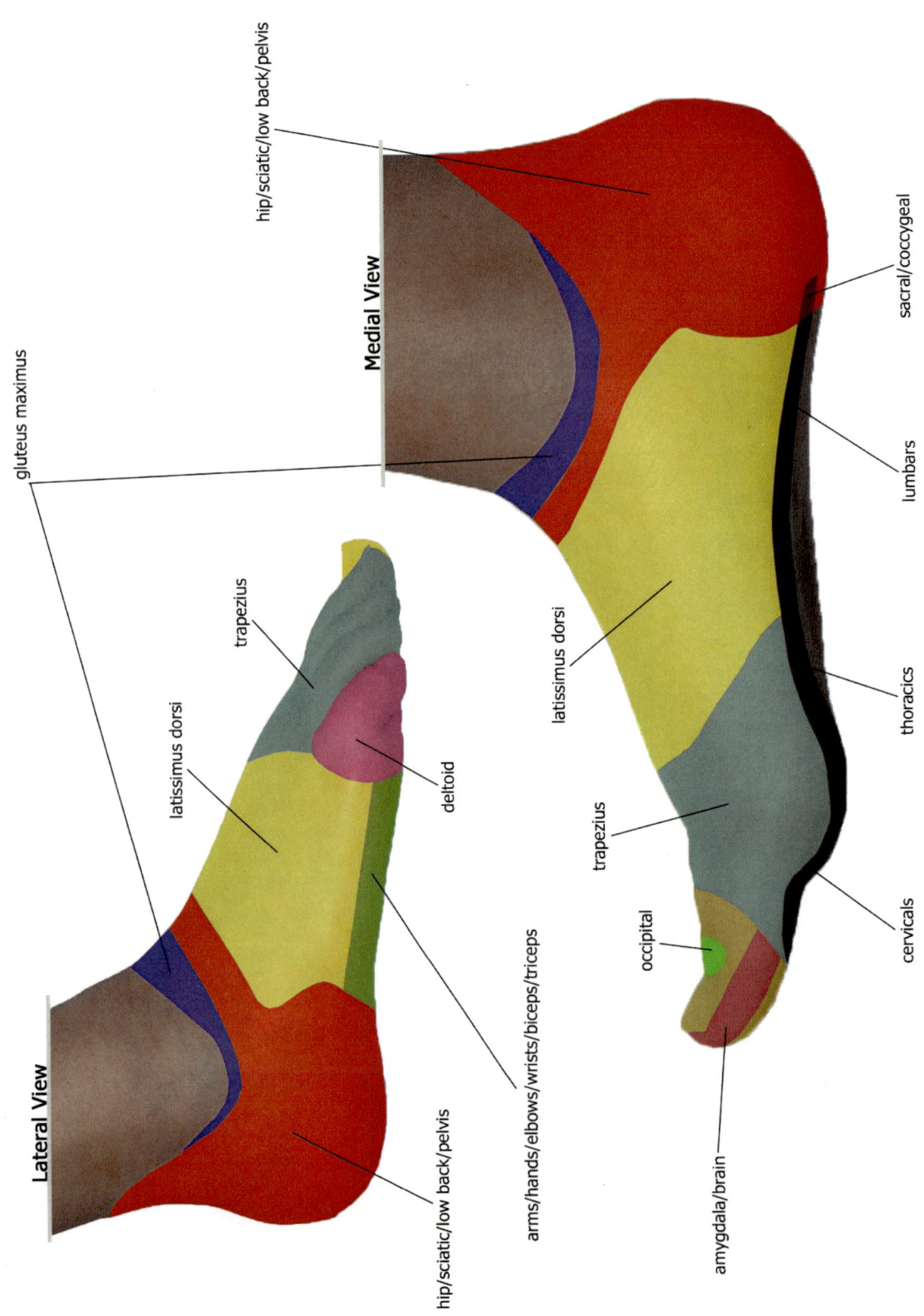

Chapter 6 – Understanding the Charts

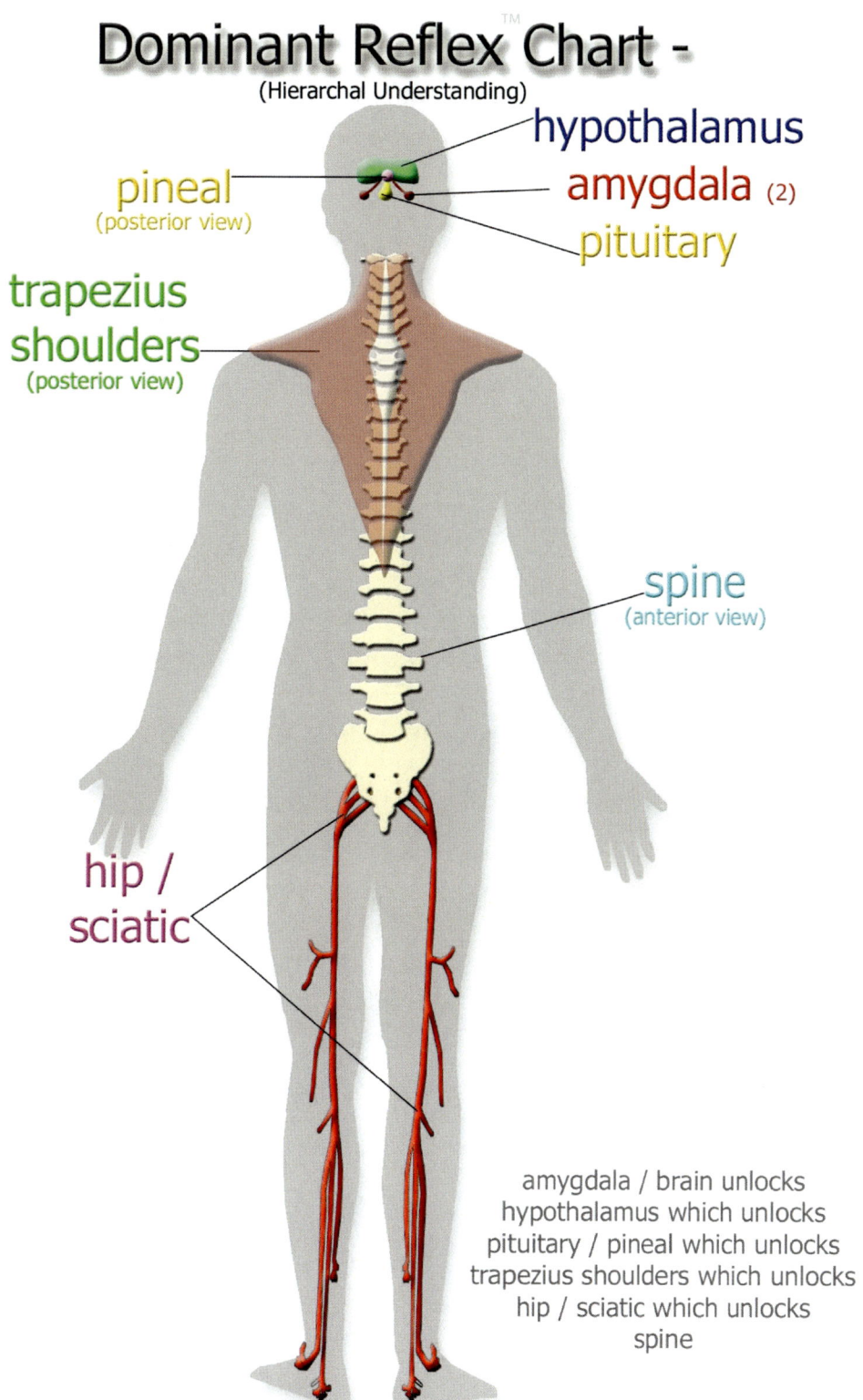

amygdala / brain unlocks
hypothalamus which unlocks
pituitary / pineal which unlocks
trapezius shoulders which unlocks
hip / sciatic which unlocks
spine

Chapter 6 – Understanding the Charts

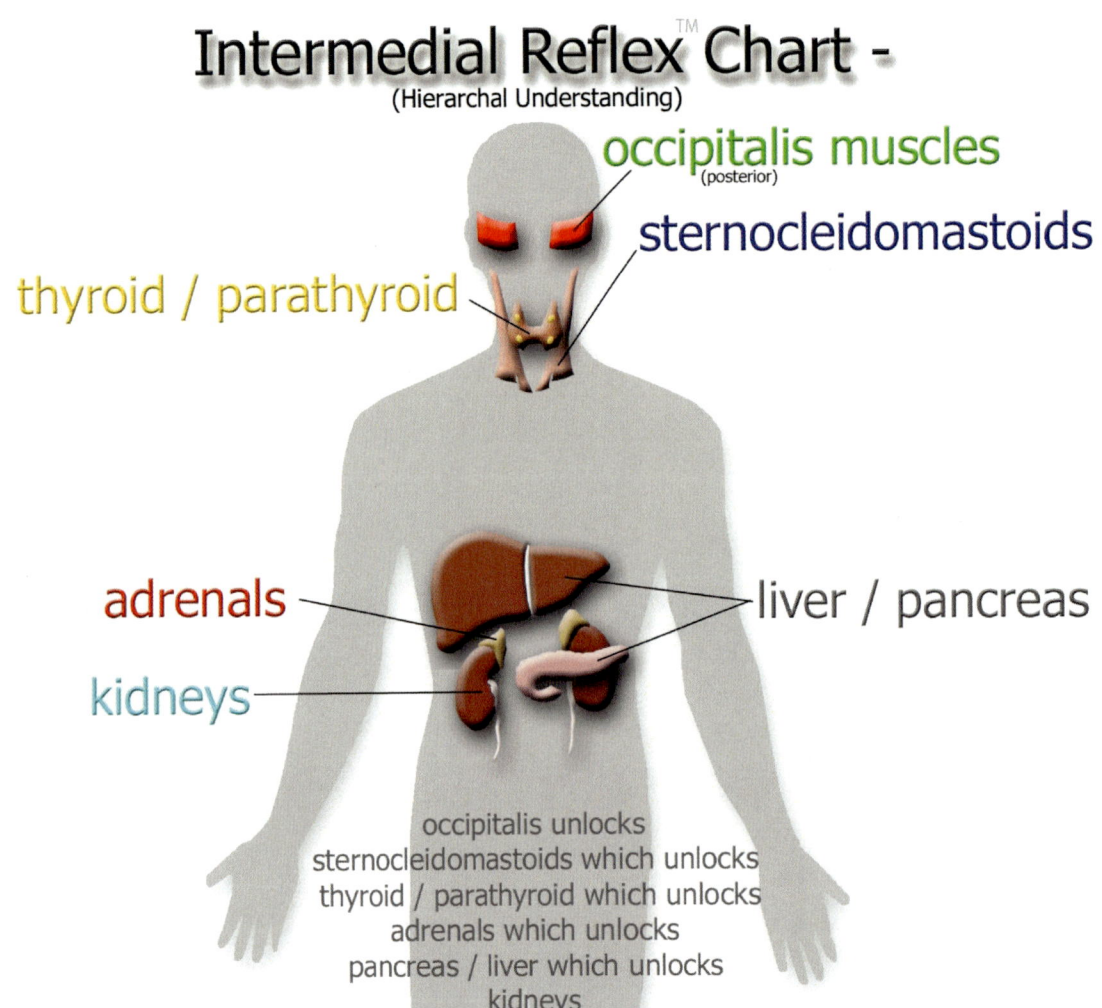

Chapter 6 – Understanding the Charts

Chapter Seven

Taking Care of Yourself and Your Equipment

Taking Care of Yourself and Your Equipment

As a reflexologist who is serious about having a long career I know that I must take care of myself and you need to take care of yourself if you'd like to practice well into your seventies like my good friend Harold Charleston.

Beside the basic staples of nutrition and exercise my suggestion to you is hand stretching briefly between treatments. There are many different ways to do this such as interlocking your fingers and turning them over and stretching them towards the ceiling. However, let me show you four important stretches that will keep your hands limber and happy for years to come.

For the purposes of these stretching exercises we'll be referring to the 'Right' hand for all images.

Dorsal Flexing of the Hand

No matter what stretch you perform, keep the arm of the hand you are stretching straight. Let's start with **dorsal flexing of the hand** (see *figure 7-1*). Sitting or standing you want your body to be centered. So sit (or stand up) straight with your shoulders square (rolled slightly back). Put your right arm out in front of you, stiff and straight. Grab the fingers of the right arm (using, of course, your left arm) with a cupping motion of your left hand. Fill your left hand with all five fingers of the right and pull back gently.

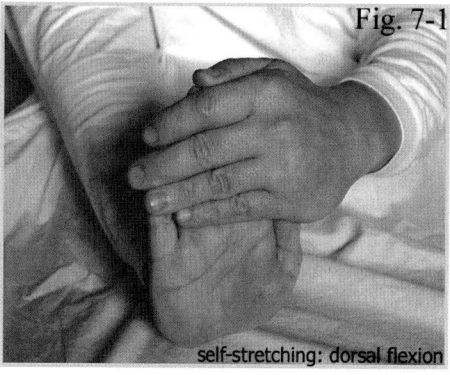
Fig. 7-1
self-stretching: dorsal flexion

You will notice a pull of the lower forearm muscles. Pull back as far as you can without injuring yourself, keeping your right hand stiff and flat while keeping your fingers together. Do not allow the elbow of the hand being stretched to collapse – keep it firm and straight. Hold for approximately 10-12 seconds. Rest for approximately the same period of time and repeat.

Plantar Flexing of the Hand

Then go right into **plantar flexing of the hand** (see *figure 7-2*) while still keeping the arm straight. Take your left hand, slide it from the plantar aspect of the hand over to the dorsal aspect of the hand being stretched and pull, cupping all the back side of the fingers and pulling them towards the body for approximately 10-12 seconds. You will feel the stretch in your upper forearm.

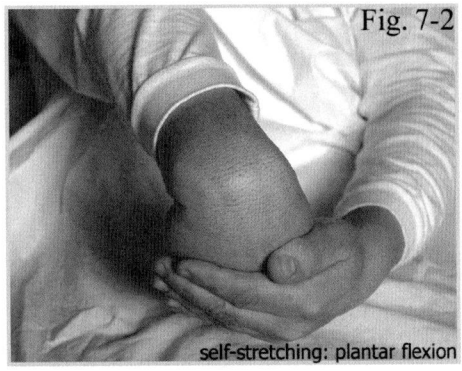

Adduction Wrist Stretch

While the arm remains straight, reach with your left hand over the top of your right wrist and place your thumb into the lateral aspect of your carpals while the fingers wrap over the top of the wrist. Now drive your thumb into the carpals as you pull and rotate the wrist medially. We use the correct term of **adduction**, meaning towards median, to refer to this movement (see *figure 7-3*).

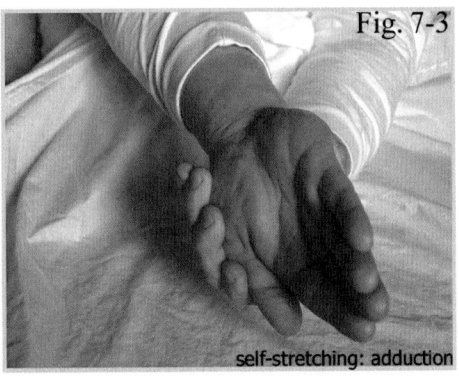

Abduction Wrist Stretch

After holding the furthest part of the stretch for 10 seconds, reverse the process by putting the left thumb into the medial part of the dorsal side of the carpals while using the other parts of the fingers to grip around the thumb. Drive your thumb into the dorsal aspect as you pull on your thumb. This movement is what we call abduction – meaning away from median (see *figure 7-4*).

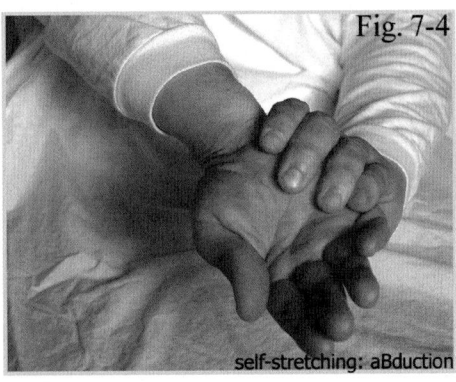

Phalanges Exercise

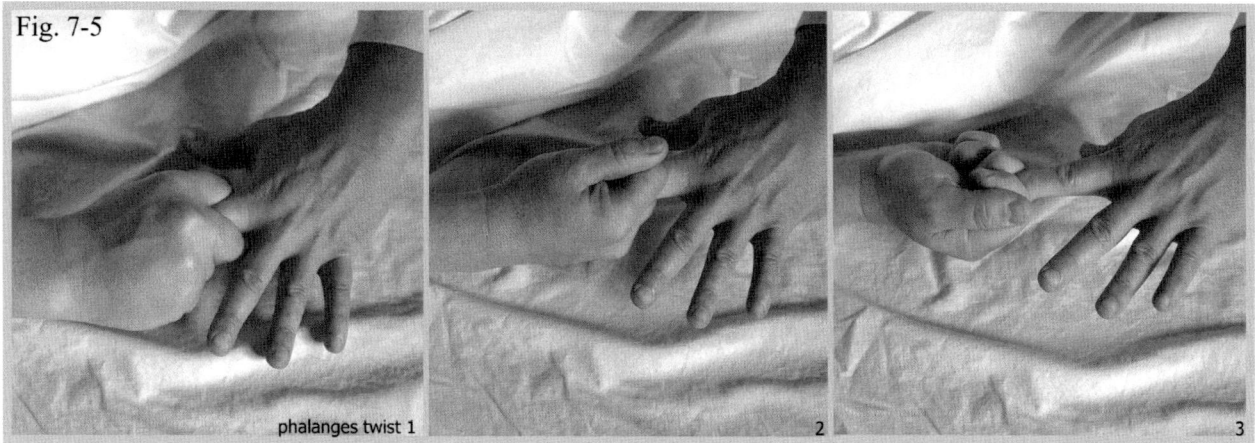
Fig. 7-5
phalanges twist 1   2   3

As I stated earlier, if you wish to stay in this business a long time, you must take care of your own hands and fingers by stretching them and keeping them mobile. A quick and simple technique for taking care of the fingers is to do what I call the 'phalanges twist'.

Simply take the index finger and second digit of the working hand and, like the hallux twist, open and wrap those fingers around the base of the finger to be worked. The pictures (see *figure 7-5*) show me working on the index finger, but you could start anywhere.

Bend your fingers at the proximal-interphalangeal joint and squeeze. Then, while pulling the finger, twist back and forth until you have made it all the way to the fingernail. This will not only stretch the finger joints but will soften the tissue increasing sensitivity and mobility.

Keep the Nails Trimmed

It is the responsibility of each practitioner to keep his or her nails trimmed and without irregularities. For those of us that are nail-biters we must remember to keep the jagged edges of the nails smooth. This way we will not cut or irritate the skin of a client.

I know what you're thinking (if you're a woman, anyway), 'I don't want to cut my long, beautiful, well-manicured nails!' If you want to be a professional reflexologist who is not accused daily of stabbing your patients, CUT YOUR NAILS!

Halitosis (Bad Breath)

Halitosis is the enemy of social interaction. I've been guilty of drinking a couple cups of my favorite organic coffee only to have forgotten to control my 'coffee-breath' as I greeted my first client of the morning. You will see their eyes widen and heads pull back as a reminder to check your breath. If you're on a low-carb diet, ketosis will give you powerful bad breath. Find a breath mint you like and keep them handy.

Cleanliness

I can't say enough about cleanliness. Nothing makes a prospective client feel so secure as a clean environment.

Make sure that you practice good grooming habits in personal care and appearance. Specifically, make sure you are showered each day and your clothes are clean and without untended tears or stains. Please don't promote your disdain for aluminum carrying deodorant products by allowing yourself to stink. If you want to use natural deodorants (which I recommend) make sure they mask any body odor. Check yourself between clients.

If the client keeps his eyes open during treatment, they will be focused on you. If you are wearing dark clothes, expect dry skin from the clients to be highly visible and take care to brush it off after treatments. You may have to spray yourself with germ spray for hygiene purposes.

If you're in the habit of constantly touching your face – make sure you keep anti-bacterial cleansers around. I use these to clean my hands between clients' visits. Keep your hair trimmed and neat. If you look professional you would receive more respect and recognition.

Some of the client's feet, even though they've cleaned them, still have oil and dirt that will collect under your nail beds. It's just a fact of the business. If this happens scrub your nails clean in the sink before seeing the next client.

In the treatment room itself, keep your carpet vacuumed and your chair wiped clean. Also have a clean head towel for the headrest for each client as well as spraying down the chair with anti-bacterial spray. Keep the room dusted and free of spiderwebs. The waiting area of your location should also present a neat and clean appearance.

Colognes

Colognes / perfumes have different effects on people. One might love a particular scent but this same scent might produce a migraine headache for another person. Since you do not know how it would affect your clients don't use it at all.

Unless you are an expert in aromatherapy, do not burn scented candles, incense or fragrant oils for relaxation for the same reason: you never know what bothers other people. It is better for the practitioner to remain scent-neutral in all regards including your deodorant.

The only rule I break pertaining to smell is this: I use Lysol™ to spray down the chair and carpet between patients' visits. Lysol™ is universally known as a germ fighter and people recognize the smell. They know the place had been cleaned and sanitized.

Equipment

My recommendation is to have a chair that the client feels no lumbar compression whatsoever when in the reclining position. It should also have a headrest. I have no financial interest in LaFuma™ chairs, but I highly recommend their 'zero-gravity' chairs for two reasons: One, it is lightweight (less than 20 lbs.). This makes it a real joy when carrying it into clients' homes or moving it to clean around. It feels almost weightless. That's ironic considering reason # 2. The chair is extremely strong. It can hold a 350 lb. man comfortably. The chair has incredible endurance. The second-to-the-last LaFuma™ chair I bought barely needed re-stringing after almost 2 ½ years of commercial use and you can do the stringing yourself. The cost of the new string is negligible.

I learned 'you get what you pay for' when the off-brand chair I bought fell apart in six months. There are some heavy duty, VERY pricey reflexology chairs out there, but for the strength, the price and ease of transport, LaFuma™ is the best.

Position your furniture so that direct sunlight from a window is not in the client's eyes. Have soft lighting and gentle instrumental music for optimally tranquil atmosphere.

Having a restroom nearby is a must when considering office space because your clients will most likely have to use it after a treatment. Check it afterwards to make sure it stays clean.

What About Music?

I do own a reflexology CD that plays soft, music interspersed with sounds of the ocean and birds chirping. Many of my clients have complimented how soothing and relaxing the sound makes them feel. Unfortunately I only have it at one of my offices but I plan on rectifying that.

Lighting

If at all possible keep the lighting low but not too low where your client may feel claustrophobic or would have to strain to see. Natural light coming through a window would be optimal – just make sure it's not shining into your client's eyes. One of my offices has bright fluorescent light overhead and there's not much I can do about it because of the way the lights are stationed for the whole building.

****

As a final note, the better the atmosphere, the more comfortable your client will be. This would make a good impression of you and a return visit is more than likely to happen.

Chapter 7 – Taking Care of Yourself & Your Equipment

Chapter Eight

Thumb-driving, Holding, Stretching and Relaxation Techniques

Chapter 8 – Thumb-driving, Holding, Stretching & Relaxation Techniques

Thumb-driving, Holding, Stretching and Relaxation Techniques

I will go over basic techniques that, when used as a foundation, should help you to become a better reflexologist.

Thumb-Driving (walking) – is the primary way a reflexologist strikes reflexes in the body. This technique uses the thumb to press, push and drive flesh in order to facilitate the reflex reaction. The angle of the thumb should be natural and the majority of the force needed to travel long planes of the foot should come from the wrist and forearm.

There are some rules that cannot be broken and then there are principles which allow for the freedom of each unique practitioner to develop their own art and skill of thumb-walking. Let's go over a couple of rules that cannot be broken:

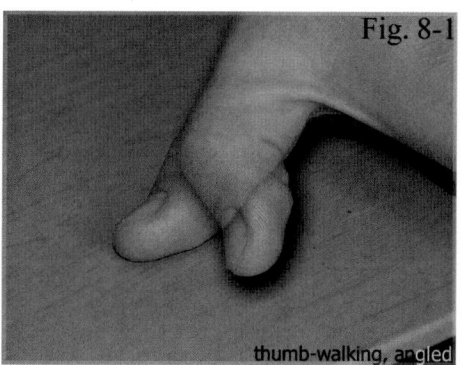
Fig. 8-1 — thumb-walking, angled

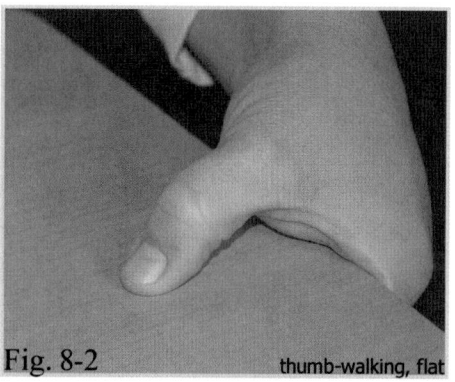
Fig. 8-2 — thumb-walking, flat

- Thumb-driving must always be in the forward motion in order to stretch each section of the skin into the flattest plane possible (one exemption of this rule would be – unless you're doing a circular pressure point such as the hypothalamus or hip / sciatic around the base of the heel). Here's what I don't want to see: as the working thumb walks in a forward motion, the practitioner relaxes and flattens the interphalangeal joint of the thumb (straightening it) – thus pulling the skin backwards (the 'inchworm effect').

  The thumb must always be bent (dorsal flexion) as you drive it forward. Use the forefingers as leverage to anchor the thumb firmly against the skin and use a combination of both wrist / forearm wrenching along with a bending of the thumb for premium reflex strike. <u>Keep the natural angle of your thumb at its most distal point in contact with the skin.</u> (see *figure 8-1*) Try to use only the full head of the

Chapter 8 – Thumb-driving, Holding, Stretching & Relaxation Techniques

thumb when crossing transverse planes (see *figure 8-2*). How much wrenching of the wrist and forearm will be up to each practitioner according to their own art and discernment. But to reiterate the law that must not be broken: no backward movement causing the loss of forward motion and the pulling back of the skin.

- Excessive plantar-flexing of the digits (toes) 2-5 is a 'no-no'. Toes naturally bend in a dorsal fashion and can even feel pleasant to the client. However, flexing the toes in the opposite direction can give your client great alarm. It gives them the sensation that you're going to break their toe. That is why you need sound training that you can only get in class to perform this maneuver. Stick to extension when trying to stretch the digits.

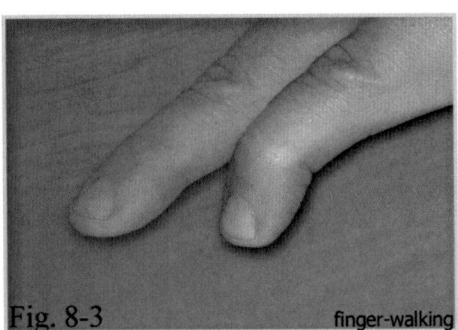
Fig. 8-3   finger-walking

Basic Finger Techniques

Using the fingers is an excellent way to reach reflexes that the thumb simply cannot. The fingers can get into tight places – such as: between, back and sides of the toes. And are excellent for reaching hip / sciatic reflexes of the ankle area. The same rules apply to finger-driving as with thumb-driving. The only exception to this is when you're working under the back side of the heel between the talus and over the calcaneus to the plantar pad. I use a dragging motion with small 'bites' while pulling for extension of the heel (see *figure 8-3*). It's more of a 'hooking' technique than a 'driving' one, really. By using this method I am still able to stretch the skin in order to reach the reflexes.

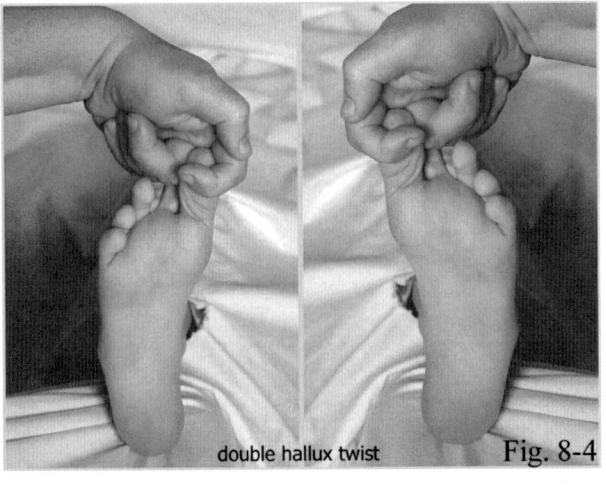
double hallux twist   Fig. 8-4

We also use the fingers to act as a vice grip, to perform the hallux twist (*see figure 8-4*) and for working the phalanges of the hands. For depth of drive for either thumb or fingers, refer to Chapters Ten, Eleven and Twelve that illustrate performing the Dominant, Intermedial and Elementary reflexes, respectively.

Chapter 8 – Thumb-driving, Holding, Stretching & Relaxation Techniques

Understanding the Length of Treatment

It is important for the reflexologist to understand when too much of a good thing can be bad for the client. I'm a firm believer that reflexes can be overstimulated which is why I'm adamantly against reflexology shoes. The constant stimulation received by the prodding of vertical protrusions in the base of the shoe drives the nervous system crazy. It will result in the brain discounting and cutting-off such stimulation from its diagnostic system because it will ascertain a malfunction of its society.

Stimulating of reflexes should grab the attention of the brain and the nervous system for special attention. But could you imagine if your friend called you every 5 minutes, 12 hours a day, 5 days a week? With the same information? You'd start ignoring your nutty friend. The brain behaves the same way, because it must discern what's imperative to sustain life function and what is NOT imperative or outright useless.

This is an important understanding with regards to the Holland Method of Reflexology. My theory is that reflexes reach a pinnacle point at around three to four strikes. It is safer to stay around three to five passes but I am certainly not dogmatic due to the uniqueness of each individual. Think of it as walking up the top of a three to four-story staircase (a pinnacle peak structure) that when you get to the top, you find out there is nothing except a giant drop-off. Working that reflex one more time is like taking that last step, where no step exists.

It works like this: Let's go back to the back-scratch illustration. Would it feel good when you ask someone to scratch your back, and the first swipe was hard, deep and fast? Of course not, that would be too alarming to the body and you would jump forward.

The superior approach would be a light scratch over the identified area with increased depth and stride between each scratch. With each subsequent scratch the recipient feels better and better...but to a point. The pinnacle comes when the sensory nerves say, 'That's enough.' That's usually the same moment the recipient pulls their shirt down and leans forward and says, 'Thanks, that's good.'

Now what was involved in the back scratch? It was nerves in the dermis that communicated to the recipient that skin cells were blocking the new growth of cellular skin and thus it needed to be removed. Once a sufficient amount of scratching was done the sensory nerves then notified the recipient that the scratches were no longer needed and that the scratching must desist as a defense mechanism to protect the integrity of the new skin. Reflexes are the same way. If attacked at the outset through high pressure the client's own defense system will jerk the foot away. It is too quick of an action for the central nervous system to relax against and just submit. This is an important point to note – that the first round of all reflexes from dominant to intermedial to elementary must be gentle. I call this 'Level One'.

How Much Pressure should I use?

There are a three levels of pressure you should become familiar with. Unfortunately, those three levels will not be the same in any practitioner. Experience, technique, and personal strength will determine what those three levels are. But you must, as a reflexologist, be able to divide your skills by three.

Level One

It's amazing how many clients you will come in contact with who will be in agony just by your performing the most basic reflexes during Level One. The reason could be two-fold. One is that the client has a lot of congestion in his feet and the nerves have not received proper blood flow in many years. The other is the entire physiological system of the client is in complete disarray and needs complete re-booting for homeostasis.

With the latter point in mind it is good to note that these individuals may be undergoing tremendous stress or are highly toxic from poor diet, medication and/or environment. Even so, do not let the client beg off from following through with the first treatment. What I would do is perform Levels One, Two and Three at the same intensity of Level One.

Level One of the Pinnacle Peak Structure is to allow the client's feet to get used to the practitioner's hands and to receive the appropriate amount of pain that will prepare them for increased pressure and discomfort on Levels Two and Three (further up the staircase). I make sure to reach ALL the reflexes during Level One and there is no particular order to how the reflexes are worked on this level. I will also incorporate a few relaxation and stretching techniques at the end of Level One to prepare the feet for Level Two.

Level Two

Level Two is where we as reflexologists get busy as we think with the hierarchal

Chapter 8 – Thumb-driving, Holding, Stretching & Relaxation Techniques

structures in mind. The first would be the dominant. I would start with the dominant chart and its reflexes at a pressure slightly higher than Level One pressure. Gauge the response of your client. If they can handle more pressure (within reasonable pain tolerance), by all means, give it to them.

A special note: In my experience, men will not always be honest about how much pain they're in because of ego. Make it very clear upfront that if they do not tell you when the pain becomes unbearable and they just 'grin and bear it' this will actually have a detrimental effect on our goals; notwithstanding they may not come back under a lame excuse when the real reason is you caused them too much pain. Also make clear that you can't feel their pain and thus, require their input to gauge the intensity of pressure you need to use. Feedback is necessary to do our job.

*I'm a very strong man who's been doing this for ten years and I can break a glass bottle with my bare hand (**see Doug's forearm muscle figure 8-5**). But that kind of pressure is reserved for the clients who are in good physical condition.*

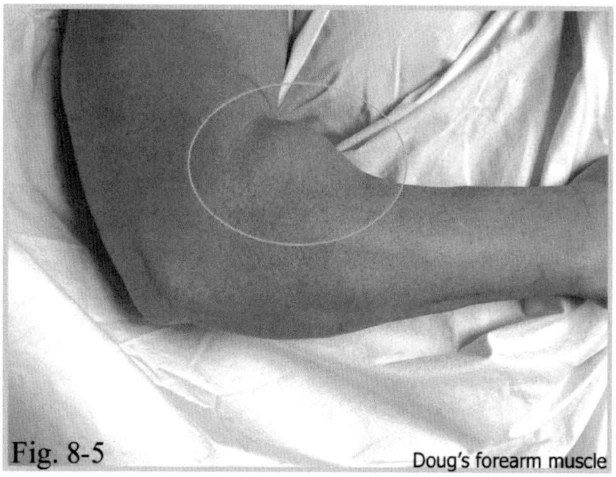

Continue with the intermedial chart and its associated reflexes followed by elementary in random, artful formation. Here's where I let my students decide what they feel is the next best reflex to strike based on their client's health and needs.

Fig. 8-5 Doug's forearm muscle

Level Three

The client now should be in the most vulnerable position for the maximum striking of the dominant reflexes followed by the other hierarchal reflexes. Remember, we've already made sufficient passes on Levels One and Two, priming them for the maximum level.

This is where good judgment is needed that seems to only come from experience. New clients may need two or three visits before I execute the type of pressure that I believe is necessary to give them the most beneficial treatment. It is at this level that I am truly in tune with the feet, the client's personality, the pain levels that are being meted out and what I believe through my own art, that I can get away with. My job is to make the brain submit and this level is where the 'fight is on'. It is after this level that I watch my client's eyes become glazed as the central nervous system responds to my wishes. In simpler terms, this is the level that I want the 'knock-out' punch to be involved in. After I'm done with this level, any subsequent passes over the reflexes should almost feel like light touch and the pain should be negligible and should feel relaxing.

Now that's a treatment that I'd be willing to pay for.

Make no mistake: this is an art that requires a tremendous amount of practice, dedication and fellow feeling for the longing to make the client feel the best they've ever felt. Quickly learn to dismiss those who will not be helped under any circumstances and who are critical of reflexology in general. This modality has changed the lives of thousands of people and as far as I'm concerned is an absolutely necessary slice in the health care pie of life.

Once the peak of the reflexes are struck, discontinue high pressure on reflexes and focus on the descending emotions and easement of stress of client. This is the peak and the going over the other side of the mountain. If a person was to continue hammering these reflexes over and over for hours on end, overstimulating them, you could imagine that at some point the brain begins to discount the alarm and actually no longer works for the issues you've presented (just like in the back-scratch illustration).

How to Gain Proper Leverage with the Holding Hand

Leverage – the perpendicular distance from the line in which a force acts upon a body to a point about which the body may be supposed to turn (according to Webster's Dictionary).

The way I look at leverage, with regards to reflexology techniques, it is how to balance the power of the holding hand with the thrust of the working hand. In most circumstances, the holding hand holds the foot in a suitable position using positional force.

The holding hand does a few things: it must stabilize the foot, it must counteract the force of the working hand and yet at the same time not crush the foot it is holding. You cannot grab the toes so hard that you crush them trying to equalize the force of the working hand.

You will learn over time how to improve on this skill and balance your powers to the

Chapter 8 – Thumb-driving, Holding, Stretching & Relaxation Techniques

point it becomes instinctive. To illustrate: Think about the art of making clay pots by hand. How you squeeze and roll your fingers will determine if the pot is shaped properly or smooshed.

Holding

The holding hand should use just the right amount of pressure to keep the foot in place so that your working hand can move across the reflex area in a stable fashion. People should be more aware of your working hand than your holding hand. Keep your elbow as well as your arm relaxed while holding the foot. This will ensure that you won't exert too much pressure in your hand grip.

Stretching

Stretching of the feet, in general, is very important to open up blood circulation in order to stimulate the nerves, release toxins and limber up the feet for greater mobility. I believe that extension movements are not only extremely safe but very effective in opening joint structures (such as tarsal, metatarsal and phalangeal conjunctions).

Using extension movements helps release synovial fluid from the joints and stretch ligaments as well as tendons. The way to do a proper extension is to become familiarized with how both hands act as levers to pull in a linear motion (in a straight line) as referenced by the larger extremity. In other words, whatever extremity you are working on must line up with the larger extremity when the extension is performed. In the following example of the Tarsal Stretch, you will notice that the foot, which is the smaller extremity, is pulled away from the leg (or the larger extremity) in a straight line.

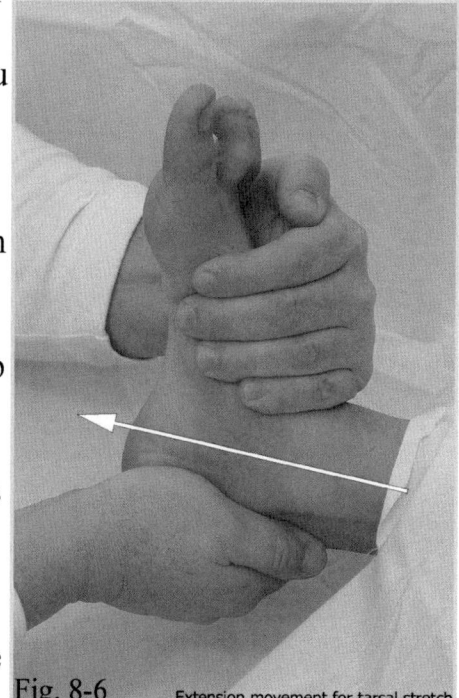

The Tarsal Stretch requires equal pressure from the top hand that lays over the dorsal part of the foot and the bottom hand that cups under the ankle. Notice in the picture (*see figure 8-6*) how the palm of the left hand is on the lateral aspect of the foot and how the fingers reach over the top and touch the medial line.

Also pay attention to how the top hand is not pulling the

Fig. 8-6   Extension movement for tarsal stretch

Chapter 8 – Thumb-driving, Holding, Stretching & Relaxation Techniques

top of the foot forward nor is it allowing it to 'fall back'. It is keeping the foot in an upright 'L' shape. The bottom hand is keeping the ankle from twisting medial to lateral. The palm of the right hand (the holding hand) finds a snug groove between the calcaneus and talus bones while the fingers reach around and find the same on the opposite side.

With a firm, strong movement, pull the foot straight back towards you, maintaining a straight line with the rest of the leg. Hold for approximately three seconds, then – as you start to ease off to let the leg contract, quickly pull again to cause maximum stretch. This 'quick pulling' lasts less than a second and is designed to catch the client off guard who may be tensing up from the movement. Afterwards, release pressure off the stretch and let the leg gently contract.

Remember the body naturally wants to defend itself and nervous clients may also. My stepfather, who is a chiropractor, deals with this daily - on how to trick the mind into relaxing at a critical moment in order to perform techniques around the body's natural defenses.

Metatarsal Stretching includes any stretching that engages mostly the metatarsal bones, surrounding muscle, and the ligaments that connect them.

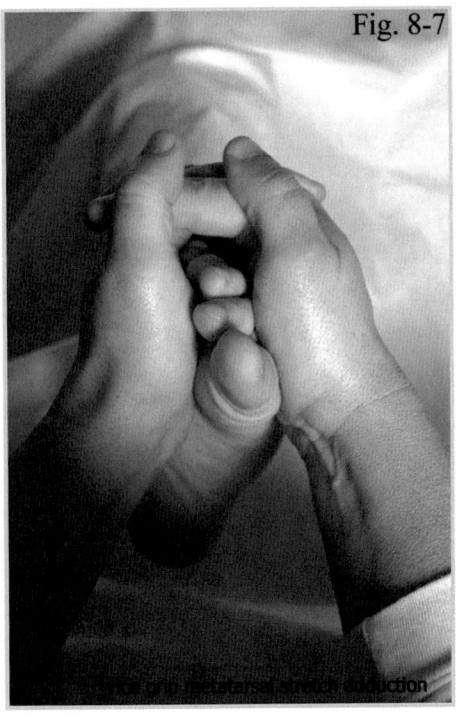
Fig. 8-7

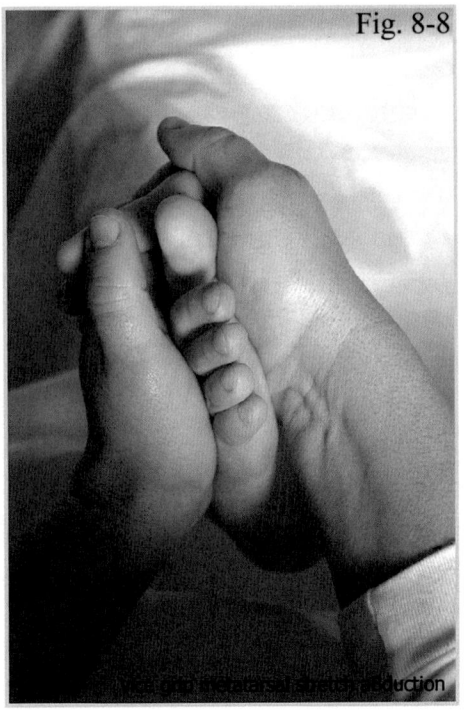
Fig. 8-8

Chapter 8 – Thumb-driving, Holding, Stretching & Relaxation Techniques

Adduction metatarsal stretch *(see figure 8-7)* is a stretch that requires the interlocking of the fingers of both hands. Place the right palm on the dorsal part of the right foot. And place the palm of the left hand on the plantar side of the foot. Slide both hands right up to the base of the phalanges while closing in your grip. Use equal pressure from both sides while you gently twist the foot medially. Once you feel the resistance becoming strong, then hold the position and do not go any further for up to 10 seconds.

Now do the opposite – **Abduction metatarsal stretch** (*see figure 8-8*) Put your left palm on the dorsal part of the foot and your right palm on the plantar side of the foot. Again, slide the hands up to the base of the phalanges while closing in your grip. Use equal pressure from both sides while you gently twist the foot laterally. As with adduction, once you feel the resistance becoming strong, hold the position and do not go any further for up to 10 seconds. Then let the foot relax.

Metatarsal Wrenching

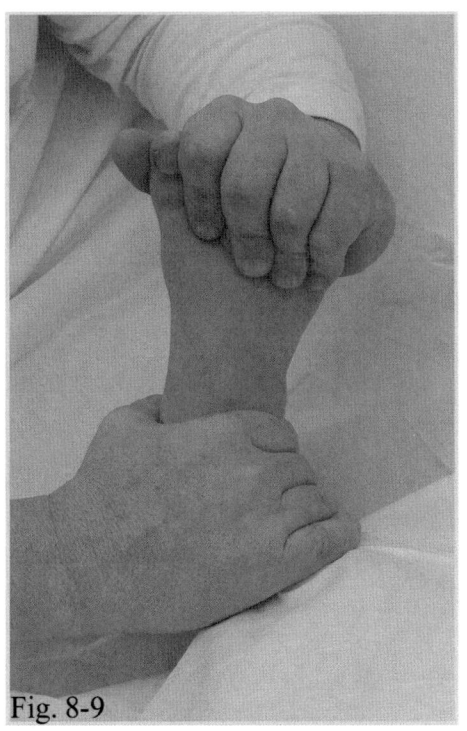
Fig. 8-9

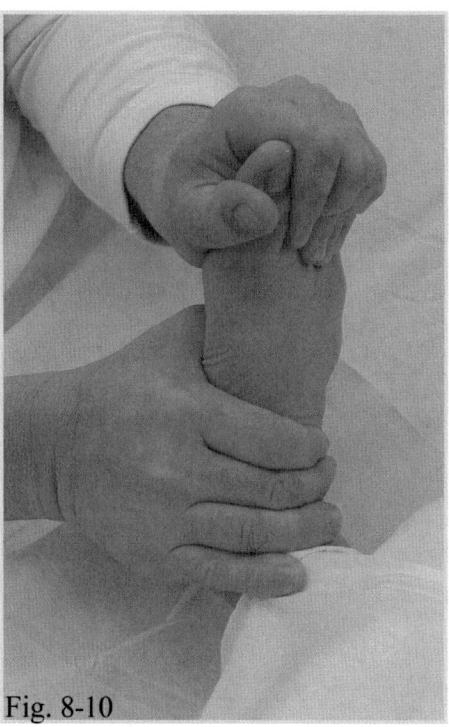
Fig. 8-10

Metatarsal wrenching is one of the best ways to really open up the metatarsal region of the foot while loosening the ankle and phalangeal bones at the same time. This particular maneuver requires a lot of strength and practice. So don't get too frustrated if you do not pick it up immediately. You will find this technique will be easier with your dominant

Chapter 8 – Thumb-driving, Holding, Stretching & Relaxation Techniques

hand on one foot versus the other. But practice both regularly to perform them fluidly.

Start by placing the right hand with the four fingers over the top of the ankle, seated in the crest between the shinbone and the metatarsals (in the U-shaped formation) the thumb should be placed underneath the plantar side. The left hand will grab the toes firmly with the palm resting on the metatarsal heads (*figure 8-9*). Begin to twist the right hand by driving the thumb into the lateral aspect of the foot while using the lateral aspect of the left hand to drive the top of the foot medially (*figure 8-10*).

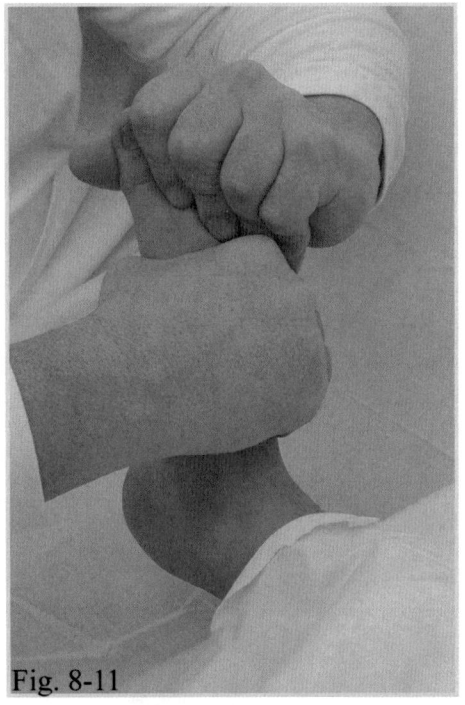
Fig. 8-11

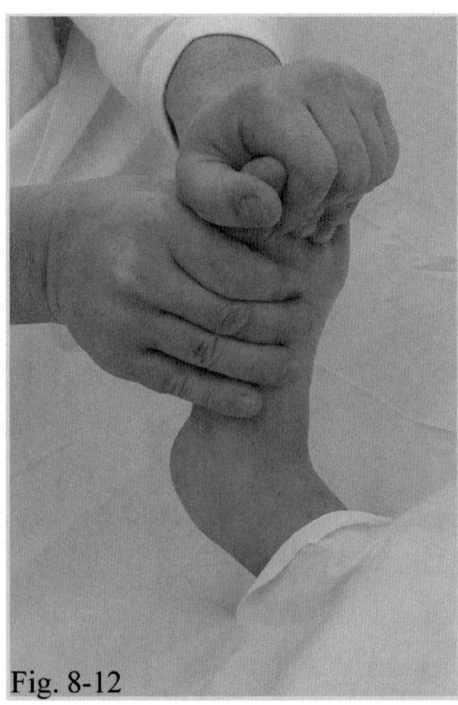
Fig. 8-12

I know it sounds weird, so I'll try to make it clearer: the bottom of the foot is moving aBduction in direction while the top of the foot is moving aDduction in direction. So both bottom and top of the foot are moving in opposite directions. As you begin twisting the hands oppositionally back and forth the only hand that will slide is the bottom hand and it will slide upward to meet the left hand (*figures 8-11 & 8-12*). How many individual wrenchings you perform up and down the foot is up to each practitioner. I personally do about three-to-four wrenchings to the top and three-to-four wrenchings on the way down.

Digital Dorsal Flexing and Achilles Stretching

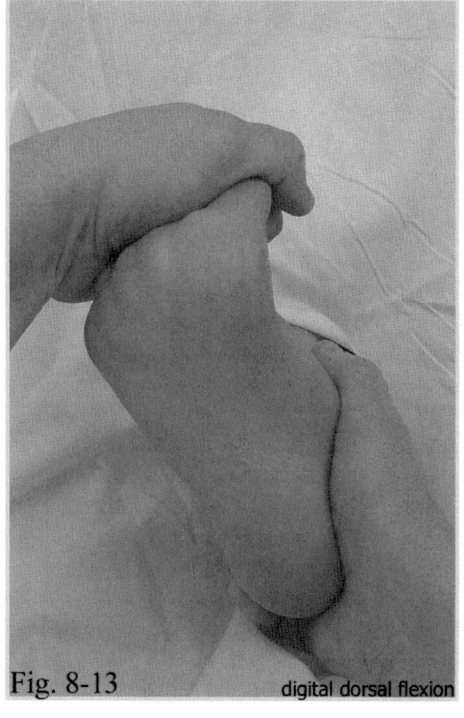

Fig. 8-13 — digital dorsal flexion

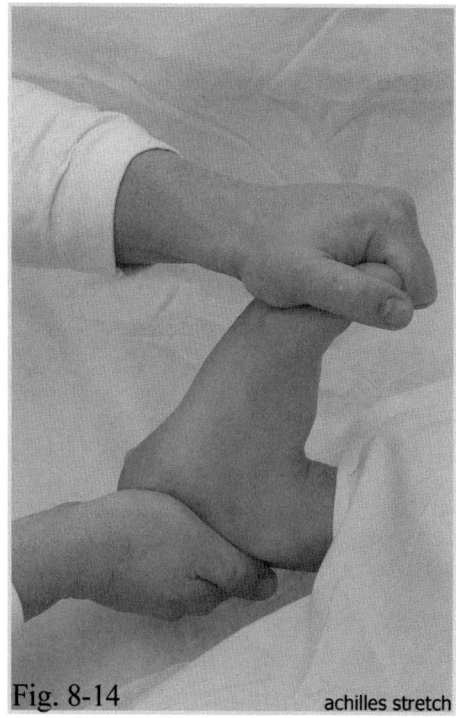

Fig. 8-14 — achilles stretch

Digital Dorsal Flexion requires you to get a firm hold with the correct holding hand (*see figure 8-13*) underneath the right ankle. Take a firm hold of the bottom of the foot, as if you were going to perform an extension movement. Now with the left hand, drive the toes back (dorsal flex) until strong resistance is felt. Take care not to overly squeeze the toes, rather use the palm of your left hand to grab hold of the digital pads. The metatarsophalangeal joints should protrude noticeably and the skin along that transverse area should be white or slightly mottled from the squeezing out of blood. This feels wonderful to the client because this stretches the phalangeal joints, the flexor hallicus longus tendon, plantar fascia as well as other tendons and muscles. Hold for 8 seconds then let the foot relax. Make sure when performing this stretch to grab hold of ALL the toes.

Achilles Stretching

Achilles Stretching is similar to digital dorsal flexing with one exception: the idea is not to stretch the toes, rather to slide the palm of the hand onto the metatarsal heads and push against those bones while pulling with the holding hand (*see figure 8-14*). The client should feel the stretch in the gastrocnemius and NOT in the toes.

Relaxation Techniques

Using relaxation techniques has many benefits during a reflexology treatment. Even though I do not focus a lot of attention on these techniques during a treatment, I will use them to soften the client at critical moments. Use relaxation methods to assist the clients' feet in getting used to your hands. A minute or so - of some stretching and relaxation before you get into the reflexes is known to put new clients at ease, and allows the practitioner access to prime reflexes that most would never let someone touch otherwise.

Many times it has been said to me that, *"No one has ever touched my feet before!"* because they are ticklish or very sensitive. Some people hate the very thought of someone touching their feet. It may be that when they were children a relative teased them by tickling their feet and chasing after them and this left emotional scars. They may also feel apprehensive because a friend told them reflexology is very painful and that they will wish they brought a leather strap to bite on. Whatever the reason, a few seconds of the subsequent relaxation techniques discussed here will do your client good by helping that tension and stress subside.

Calcaneus Rocking

Calcaneus rocking is an excellent way to loosen up the tarsals while at the same time resting the hands of the practitioner. This particular exercise uses the weight of the foot to sling the core of the foot from side-to-side allowing the tarsals to freely move and articulate from one another.

After forming two clenched fists (*see figure 8-15*), palms down, allow the heel to rest gently into the medial grooves of each fist (the 'groove' that is formed by the thumb and index finger, contracted). You will feel the heel of the foot fit snugly in the saddle of both hands. It should be very comfortable and feel natural. Make sure not to turn the joint of the index finger inward. Also, temper the intensity of the thumb's penetration into the heel so you do not lose control over the foot. In order to 'rock the foot' from side-to-side, simply raise one hand slightly higher than the other; then, lower that hand while raising the other hand in a gentle rocking motion. It helps to keep the foot elevated – slightly off any subsurface.

Fig. 8-15 calcaneus rocking

Chapter 8 – Thumb-driving, Holding, Stretching & Relaxation Techniques

Hand Drill

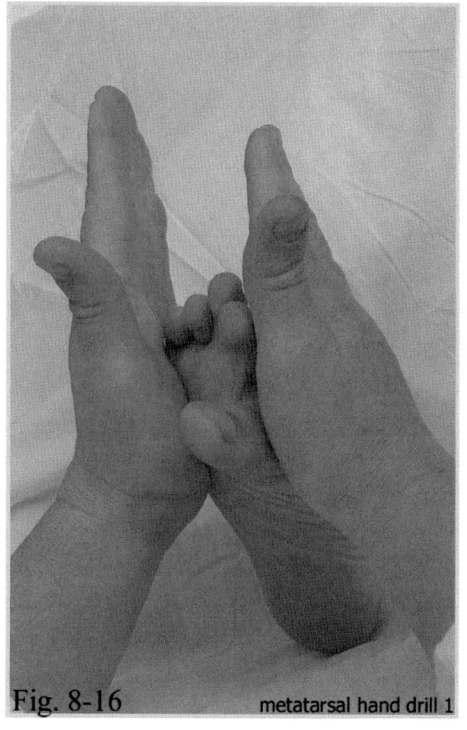

Fig. 8-16 metatarsal hand drill 1

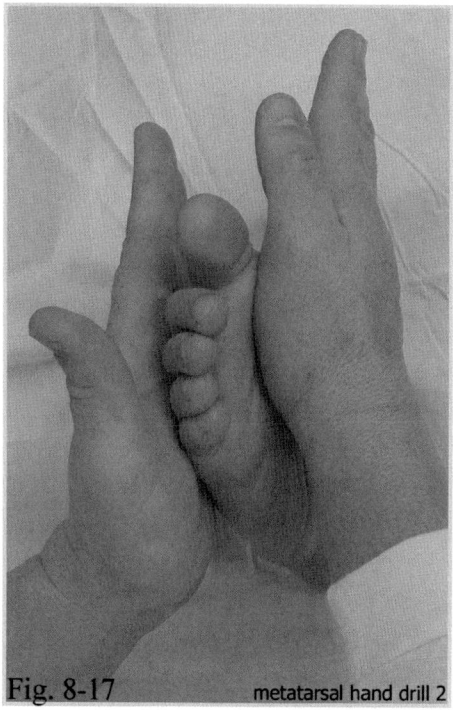

Fig. 8-17 metatarsal hand drill 2

An ancient method of fire-starting is the 'hand drill' method. The act of making a hand drill is the rubbing of two sticks together over tiny pieces of dry tinder to make a smoldering ember that, once fanned, can start a fire. We don't want to start a fire with the foot but the hand drill illustration is an excellent way to describe this relaxation technique which is designed to loosen the entire foot and break down its defensive measures.

To perform this technique correctly, the practitioner must use the right amount of gripping force coupled with the relaxation of the wrists and forearm muscles. With both thumbs straight up and fingers extended, place the plantar pad of the left hand on the lateral part of the right foot (*see figures 8-16 & 8-17*) where it meets the 5th metatarsal head. Place the plantar pad of the right hand on the medial side of the right foot where it meets the 1st metatarsal head. Now move your hands rapidly back and forth as if trying to start a fire with a hand drill. Keep your hands relaxed as you apply pressure from the plantar pads of both hands.

Metatarsal Wave

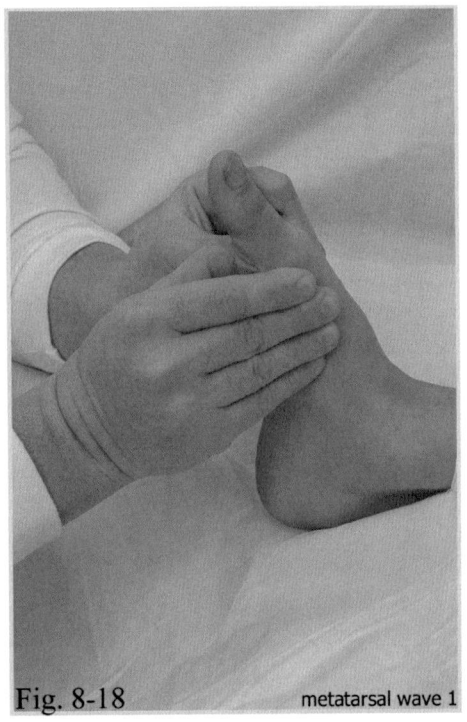

Fig. 8-18 metatarsal wave 1

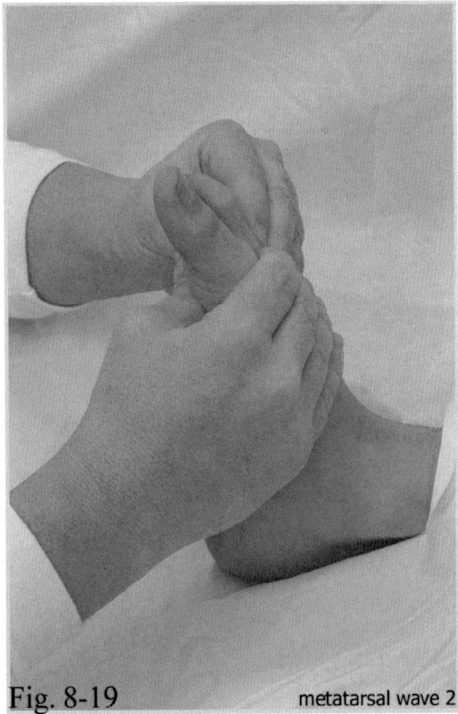

Fig. 8-19 metatarsal wave 2

The metatarsal wave relaxation technique is probably one of the most difficult techniques to master. It requires just the right amount of pinching force, compression and torquing from the thumb and forefingers than any other technique. Even though I do not focus my treatment on relaxation techniques (as I believe the therapy is through the striking of reflexes – thus the relaxation comes after the treatment) my clients have informed me that this is one of their absolute favorite movements.

The starting position is the left hand over the lateral aspect and the right hand over the medial aspect of the right foot. Both thumbs engage the metatarsal heads from the plantar aspect and the fingers pin and hold between metatarsals on the dorsal position.

Start by driving the right thumb into the right foot's metatarsal heads (adduction) while the wrist torques and

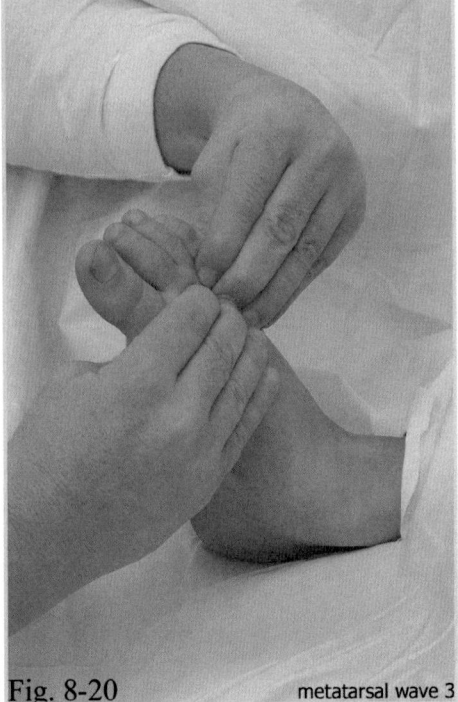

Fig. 8-20 metatarsal wave 3

follows. Once resistance is felt at the end of the right-hand torque, do the same with the left hand. Drive the thumb into the metatarsal heads (adduction) and the wrist follows. This forces a bow-shaped formation that cocks the 'whip' (*see figure 8-18*) – because there is a whip-like motion that is made. The transverse dorsal aspect of the foot should be extended or rounded.

The torquing of the right hand should remain strong as the deflection of the left hand is forced back to a lineal position (*see figure 8-19*). Allow the left hand to extend past the lineal position so that the lateral part of the foot extends past the transverse plane forcing what appears to be a bow in the the plantar region of the metatarsophalangeal conjunction (*see figure 8-20*). The right hand now torques in the opposite direction with the forefingers driving into the dorsal aspect of the metatarsal region. This whips the left hand back around to the lineal position.

Just continue to repeat this process over and over until you have a comfortable wave moving medial-to-lateral. The wave should be medial-to-lateral no matter what foot you are working on. In simpler terms we are trying to make a wave-like action mimicking waves in water bringing relaxation to the client. It also improves flexibility in the transverse region of the foot. Make sure not to squeeze too tightly with your thumb and forefingers so that you don't cause unnecessary discomfort, undermining the relaxation technique.

Hanging the Saddle

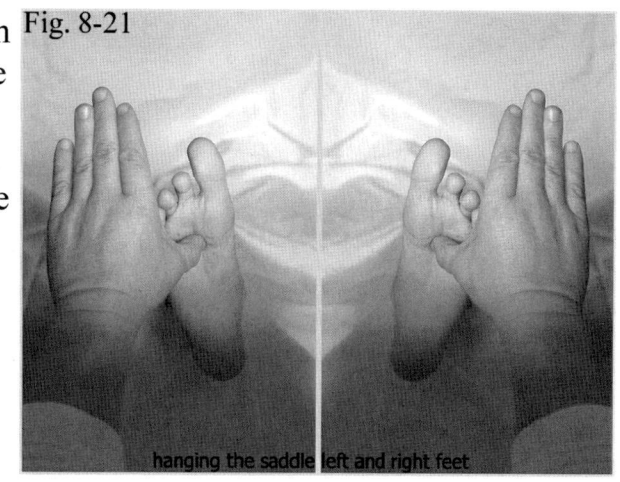

Fig. 8-21

hanging the saddle left and right feet

When you are finished with the entire session there is one relaxation technique that tells the client the treatment is over and it's time to really relax. This technique requires strength of the thumb and forearm muscles so don't be too hard on yourself if you can't hold it for very long in the beginning.

With your thumbs, find the 'saddle' just underneath the center of the transverse pad where the metatarsal heads protrude (*see figure 8-21*). You'll feel a soft spot that lies just underneath the transverse muscle that lines the base of these heads. Hook your thumbs in that saddle, while straightening your forefingers outward above the toes. Lift

Chapter 8 – Thumb-driving, Holding, Stretching & Relaxation Techniques

the feet gently just above the subsurface you are working on until you feel the weight of the feet on your thumbs. The feet should hang on your thumbs, thus the term 'hanging the saddle'.

While holding this position (approximately 1 – 2 minutes) slowly let down the feet until they're no longer hanging on your thumbs but gently resting against them. It is not uncommon to see the client sigh and deeply relax at the very end of this technique.

****

Now that you've got the hand of these important techniques, we're going to spend some time getting ready to administer the reflexology treatment.

Chapter 8 – Thumb-driving, Holding, Stretching & Relaxation Techniques

Chapter Nine

Getting Ready to Administer a Reflexology Treatment

Getting Ready to Administer a Reflexology Treatment

Preparing Mentally for Client & Greeting

Most likely the client was referred to you by a friend or family member or colleague. On rare occasions, through advertisement. However they got there, they're there. No doubt they're apprehensive about the first time meeting with you. Think about it. Even though they love their family members or friends (and trust them) they don't know you personally or the environment they're stepping into - which is also new. This is a shock to the normal system because human nature likes what's familiar.

I do not require the clients to write their medical history, diet or general conditions as I did in the beginning. My philosophy has changed on this over the years. I do, however, expect the client to give me feedback as to whether the reflexology treatment helped them in any way, shape or form. That is the proof that reflexology works, not the act of trying to treat a specific illness. It is the client's feedback that motivates me to improve as a reflexologist.

Their testimonies should inspire you to work their entire systems for the benefit of their whole body and not get side-tracked by a specific issue. I found that people that have come in for a specific problem end up telling me that reflexology helped a little bit in the area of original concern and then go on to share that reflexology helped in other ways they had not anticipated and IT becomes their primary focus. They always seem quite fascinated as to how well a single treatment of reflexology had on their constitution. It was the same way for me.

As far as **record-keeping** is concerned: a name, address and contact number are sufficient for client data. If you want to jot down notes about the client then keep files. You may also want to track each visit so as to have a good idea of how often they see you which will help in a two-fold way: one is that you can make recommendations as to their needs for treatment and the other is for marketing purposes (for more information refer to Chapter Fifteen on 'Business and Ethics').

When I did keep detailed experiences (see Chapter Fourteen 'Observations' for more information), which I've added to this book for comparisons, it seemed necessary to take detailed notes. After all – I was trying to discover how reflexology worked. However, since reflexologists cannot diagnose or treat for a specific illness, I felt there was no need to be forewarned of clinical issues that are simply not my concern. If the client so chooses to reveal facts about their health (always with the understanding that it is confidential) then that is their decision. I share whatever information I have on the subject with the added understanding that I am NOT their physician and my words are strictly my opinion as if I was a caring friend.

Make that clear to your client in the beginning. For example, you will never tell them to get off medications that have been prescribed by their doctor. You may personally feel anathema towards Big Pharma (and let's face it, who in holistic medicine doesn't?) but telling the client to adjust their 'meds' can mean serious injury to the patient who is under someone else's care.

Greeting - At First Sight

Try to meet the client standing upright with a handshake and a smile. Remember, they're nervous and whatever we can do to put them at ease will help. It's interesting to note my experience with every single one of my new clients. I bring a client into my office and I point to the center of the room and say, *"There's your chair."* I watch the client's eyes scan the full spectrum of seating arrangements around the room with the recliner dead center and hear them say, *"which one is mine?"* Even though the reclining chair sits dead center and common sense would dictate THAT'S the chair they sit in (not the stool the practitioner sits on or a bench for a family member) they still ask, *"which one is mine?"*

These are very intelligent people that are thrown off for a bit because of anxiety of the situation. Their mind is moving fast ahead and they're not thinking about the direction I just gave them. Do you remember when you received your first treatment? You may have had thoughts like these going through your mind:

'What's the treatment going to be like?'
'Did I wash my feet?'
'What is he going to think of my feet?'
'Will he be repelled by them because he thinks they're ugly?'

Or if they've been browbeaten by a friend or relative they may think: *'I know this is a stupid waste of time but I just gotta get through this so I can get my friend or relative off my back.'* You'll know this type. They roll their eyes or are very curt when you ask them questions. You feel like you're interrogating them and they probably feel interrogated.

They also may be thinking about a serious condition that is within themselves that they don't want to reveal to you but their hopes are strong that you and your modality may be the real answer. These reasons and many others are why your greeting and intent statement must be clear.

Intent Statement Explained

I make sure to stand next to them as they sit in the chair. That way I can adjust the headrest as I go over some simple facts. Do not make yourself comfortable until your client is. It's impossible to carry on a conversation with someone struggling to get comfortable. It's YOUR chair and YOUR room so help them get comfortable.

As the client takes off their shoes and socks and lays back I move to the fore and ask them how they're feeling. I listen carefully to their concerns or skepticism in the most sincere way because I am truly interested in people. Once those pleasantries are over, I go into my statement.

"Have you ever had a reflexology treatment before?" If the answer is yes, then you may say, *"Good, I hope I can meet your expectations. I'm glad that you already have knowledge of this holistic therapy so that we can get right to work and get you the treatment you need. How long since your last treatment?"* If they respond, *"It's been longer than 6 months,"* than tell them it may feel like starting over for the first time. Let them know that you are a high-pressure reflexologist and your goal is to strike as many reflexes as possible during the 20-25 minute treatment.

Some reflexes require deep acupressure techniques and can create a higher level of pain. Follow with, *"The deeper I can go, the better it is for you. However, I do not want you to be in so much pain that you fly out of the chair. I like to use a **scale of 1-10 for a reference to pain**, '1' is like I'm 'tickling' your feet and '10' would be like driving a nail through it. If we can stay around '5' then I know we're doing the best we can to reach the dominant reflexes without causing you too much discomfort that you may never want to get treated again."*

Make it clear to your client that reflexology is a form of therapy not to be confused with standard massage used for relaxation only. We're not sadists trying to cause unnecessary pain, but I believe that through pain we reach the dominant reflexes that unlock the entire human physiological system. My clients tell me that they feel cheated when they don't feel pain. I've been accused of not using the same pressure as in the beginning treatments. That's funny because we know as reflexologists that the more treatments they receive correlates to better health and thus there is less pain response from the nervous system.

Isn't it interesting that the first four or five treatments bring about complaints of pain and *'when will it end'* and *'just feel good'* but subsequently months later, they complain about NOT receiving pain and it feeling too much like a general massage. This is **what led me to a critical understanding** that despite the fact that clients complain about pain, the homeostasis needs that are derived through the nervous system supersedes our general comfort zone and the body understands what's good for it.

Pain makes people feel better with regards to reflexology and the autonomic system. Sound crazy? Not to the experienced reflexology client. They realize, as I do, that pain is a qualifier and a response that proves reflexology is actually working within the system construct. There should always be some congestion resulting in pain due to our imperfection or our level of activity. This does not mean that there is something seriously wrong because pain exists, rather it is an issuance of the need for internal reminders through this external diagnostic mechanism (foot reflexes). Just like putting a note on the refrigerator as a reminder of responsibilities of the day, so too, the reflexology treatment acts as a series of notes prodding the body to maintain homeostasis; pain is just that – the note.

If the client states that this is his or her first time visit, then you might say, *"What you're about to experience today has been experienced by hundreds of thousands of people throughout the earth for the last few thousand years. It is a form of holistic therapy designed to help your body relax and normalize. There will be pain during the treatment. How is your pain tolerance?"* Follow this with what was mentioned above about the pain scale, etc.

Be Careful of What You Say

I thought I would add a couple of warnings here before getting into inspection and treatment. During treatment this may come up and I've touched on it briefly above. However it must be emphasized:

How would you handle a situation when a client tells you they want to quit taking their medication? Acknowledge to them that it is a fine goal but they should not do it without discussing it with their doctor who prescribed the medication. Remember that reflexologists are not medical practitioners and by law, are prohibited to prescribe any type of medication. In the same token, they cannot advise patients to stop taking their medications. The only advice they can give the patients is for them to discuss with their doctor their desire to stop their medication and try alternative treatments that seem to be helping them. I can't beat this horse enough. Never tell a patient to stop taking medications.

'Will reflexology cure (insert whatever their complaint is here)?' The answer to this is, *"There are no cures and reflexology is not unique in this regard."* Be firm with this statement – no equivocating no matter how much YOU believe in reflexology, because you must make it clear that reflexology is an aid to helping the body be the best it can be. It certainly cannot go outside those parameters.

I always tell the client, *"Give me three tries to see if your general state of health improves over those three visits. And if it corrects a problem you hoped for, that's a bonus."* By explaining this to your client you are letting them know that you cannot predict an outcome, nor give them any false hopes as to how their body will react to the treatment. Many unprofessional holistic therapists will use 'snake-oil sales' in hopes of repeat business. Our repeat business comes from results.

Oils and Lotions

Succinctly put, we do not use oils and lotions. The reflexologist must make a pure contact of his thumb and fingers to the skin of the foot of the client. Oils would cause the hands to slide making it impossible to stretch the dermis for reflex strikes. Leave the oils and lotions to the masso-therapists; that is their area of experience.

If the client has pre-lotioned her feet simply wipe them off with a towel. Don't be too concerned; it just takes an extra minute. Let them know to refrain from applying lotion next time.

Beginning Treatment

We start with **inspecting the feet**. By now your hands are clean, the client is ready in the reclining position, with his shoes and socks off and you're comfortable on your own perch. First, for whatever reason, I start with the left foot. It doesn't matter which one you start with, it's just a habit with me. I look between the toes, the nail beds, the dorsal aspect and the sides of the ankle bone to see if there are any cuts, scrapes, bruising or

Chapter 9 – Getting Ready to Administer a Reflexology Treatment

other abnormalities that could affect the treatment process. I look for corns, bunions, swelling on the interphalangeal joints, ingrown toenails, fungal infections, weeping sores, etc. (Athlete's Foot is a condition that prohibits a treatment. See Chapter Four 'Conditions of the Feet' for a more in-depth discussion on Athlete's Foot).

Remember, your clients may not even be aware of injury to themselves and you might be the first one that points it out to them under inspection (this is not inconceivable, especially with diabetics dealing with neuropathy). As I grab hold of the foot for the first time I ask the client two very important questions, *"Have you had any broken bones in your feet recently?"* and *"Have you had any sprain / strains along your ankle, calf or anywhere else in the lower extremity?"* See also Chapter Five 'Conditions of the Toes' with regards to working on feet and toes with injuries.

****

Now that introductions are complete and the client and you are prepared mentally, it is time to commence treatment.

Chapter 9 – Getting Ready to Administer a Reflexology Treatment

Chapter Ten

Hierarchal Treatment:

The Dominant Reflexes

Hierarchal Treatment – Dominant Reflexes

In this chapter we will discuss how to perform the Dominant reflex techniques and an explanation as to how these reflexes affect the hierarchy and value to the entire physiological association.

Amygdala / Brain – The Most Dominant Reflex

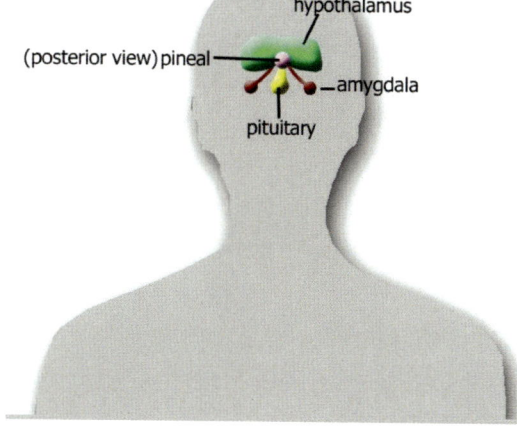

The **amygdala** is an almond-shaped structure in the brain; its name comes from the Greek word for "almond". There are actually two amygdalae. Each amygdala is located close to the hippocampus, in the frontal portion of the temporal lobe of the brain.

The latest science shows that the amygdala performs a primary role in the processing and memory of emotional reactions. The amygdala has a wide range of connections with other brain regions, allowing it to participate in a wide variety of behavioral functions such as the responsibility for activation of adrenaline, dopamine, norepinephrine, epinephrine and serotonin.

As I stated in Chapter One, if someone comes bursting into your room at night, wakes you up and points a gun at your head, you would instantly find one of the purposes of your amygdala. Some people, under great stress during an accident, have been able to lift a car off a small child with their bare hands. The amygdala can instantly communicate the need to flood the body with adrenaline in order for the entire system to engage in 'fight-or-flight'.

It also has been known to be the 'mental block' in individuals who cannot overcome Post Traumatic Stress Disorder. For some reason, the amygdala holds onto emotional memories even to one's detriment. Some that experience panic attacks, which for no reason can strike an individual at any time and cause great distress, are unaware what part of their brain is responsible for this.

Others may hold all their emotional pain and stress within themselves without expressing it openly because of the apparent control they 'appear' to exert over their amygdala.

We all know individuals like this who would never cry in public even if someone close has died - controlling their emotions using some sort of mental exercise. Their upbringing may have contributed to this; not being allowed to feel emotionally safe enough to show their emotions.

Some have been trained through martial arts or through other meditation programs to overcome general anxiety and fear that the average person deals with every day. Their mind behaves more instinctively from their training and they're less likely to react abnormally under duress.

Have you seen the videos of the individuals who stand frozen while a violent crime happens right in front of them? Comments from other individuals would follow:

'Why didn't they run?'

'Why did he just stand there?'

'Why didn't she do something?'

The reason they didn't react 'properly' is because their body was flooded with adrenaline from the adrenal glands. The adrenaline rushes in and locks all the muscles down as they contract and the person appears frozen. Their heart rate soars as the body begins to breath hard and sweat profusely. Their amygdala response had not been trained on how to deal with such a stressful situation. After all, most of us do not want to mentally prepare for the worst in life.

But, you must admit, a scientific view of the amygdala response is intriguing and this is why it peaked my interest (as to how this blocking mechanism might affect the entire association of all body members on a more minor level). Could it be that the amygdala holds the key to our improved health? I believe it does and the results I have achieved in the field have proven such.

Whatever the case, it is my belief that this is the greatest, **single most important reflex** for starting the healing process towards homeostasis that we humans have. Time and time again I have seen individuals that seem emotionless begin to cry fervently after I've

Chapter 10 – Hierarchal Treatment: The Dominant Reflexes

reached this reflex effectively. The statements they make might be:

"I don't know why I'm crying right now. I never cry."
"This is so strange, I can't keep the tears from pouring out of my eyes."
"What just happened to me? I feel so bizarre inside. I can't explain the feelings I have right now."

Others simply walk away from the treatment with glazed eyes, which I refer to as the "reflexology buzz" (my step-dad and I love that 'buzz' but we're used to it). It's as if they seem intoxicated as they struggle to put on their shoes and walk out of the office.

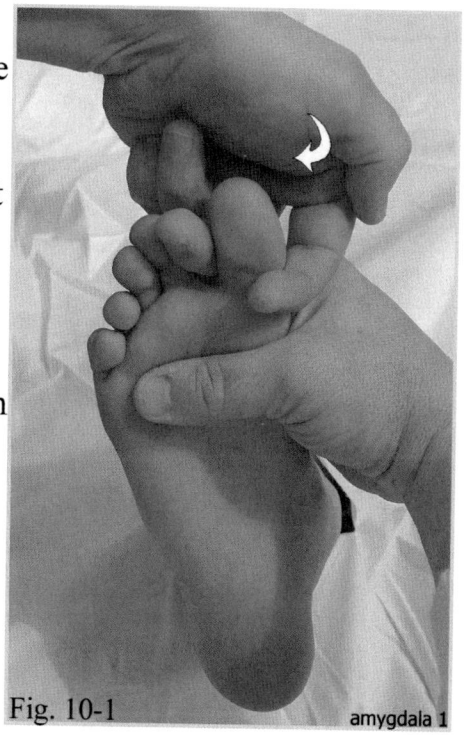

Fig. 10-1 amygdala 1

It is prudent as a professional reflexologist to take note of this reaction and give the client a few minutes and the instructions to sit down for a short while (preferably in your waiting area) to get their bearings. I've had some clients come close to injuring themselves as they get out of the chair from a loss of balance due to their fogged mental state. So stand close by them while they leave your treatment room, asking them if they are okay.

Generally they will smile, sigh and stand fully erect with shoulders broadly spaced as they report a good feeling.

In my opinion, the amygdala is the **most dominant reflex** of the entire human system because it will dominate all systems of the body if it so chooses. It unlocks emotion and relieves all tension and stress due to anxiety.

The amygdala sends impulses to the hypothalamus directly for important activation of the sympathetic nervous system, handles emotional trauma and stress, as well as expressions of fear.

If you want your clients to feel the best that they can be, make sure to make this reflex the top priority.

Brain

Nothing about the human body compares to the complexity of the brain. Your brain, along with the spinal cord and peripheral nerves make up the most multifarious control and processing system probably known to man.

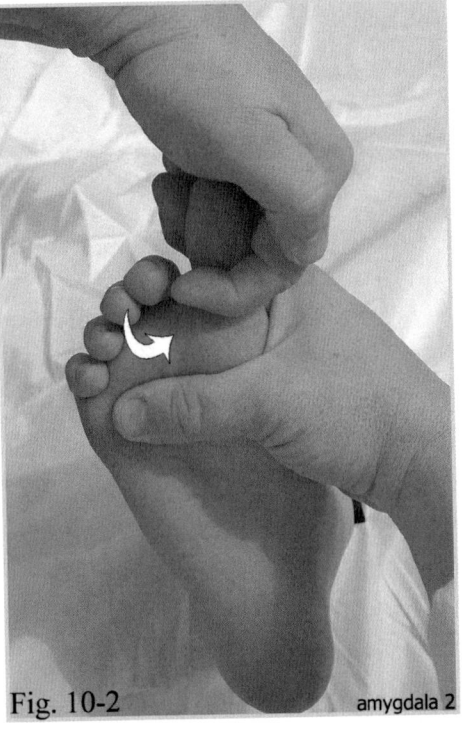

Fig. 10-2   amygdala 2

The brain is responsible for performing processes involving: motor control, all physiological needs, visual processing, auditory processing, sensation, learning, memory and emotions. You use your brain for: reasoning, falling in love, making decisions, performing in athletics – from walking to figure skating in complexity, or with such importance as an inborn conscience that tells you right from wrong. It is also important to note that we, as reflexologists, use the nervous system – which cannot do without the brain to detect issues throughout the body through the striking of reflexes.

Some brain basics:

- The brain is separated into two hemispheres: the right hemisphere that controls the left side of the body and the left hemisphere which controls the right side of the body.
- Twelve pairs of cranial nerves receive all communication from the body for the performance of functions.
- Four lobes make up the cerebrum: the frontal lobe (anterosuperior), the parietal (**per**-ree-et-ul) lobe (superior to the temporal lobe and posterior to the frontal lobe), the temporal lobe (inferior to the parietal) and the occipital lobe (posteroinferior to the other lobes).
- The cerebellum sits posteroinferior to the cerebrum.
- The brain stem sits in the most inferior position and all signals pass through it to and from the brain.

Chapter 10 – Hierarchal Treatment: The Dominant Reflexes

Performing the Amygdala / Brain Reflex Technique

This particular technique requires a gripping of the lateral aspect of the index finger with the medial of the 3rd digit between the proximal and distal interphalangeal joints.

Place the four fingers over the dorsal aspect of the right foot with the holding hand. Keep the thumb over the metatarsal heads. Your palm should be on the medial aspect of the right foot. With your other hand, split the index and 3rd digit apart while curling the distal phalanges so that a claw-like grip can be made at the very base of the hallux (*see figures 10-1 & 10-2*).

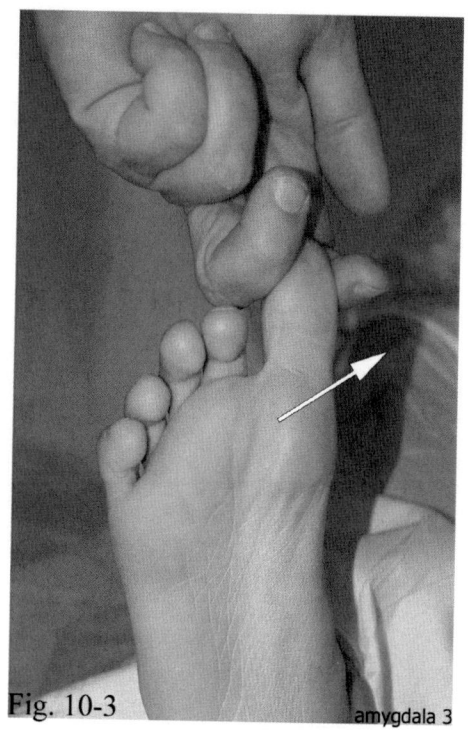
Fig. 10-3

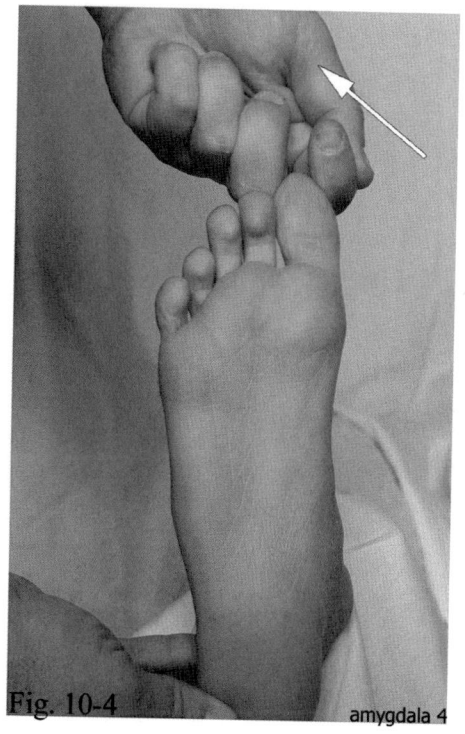
Fig. 10-4

Begin to squeeze and apply pressure at the base while slowly twisting the hand, not the fingers, medial to lateral (back and forth) all the way to the tip of the big toe. When you get to the top of the hallux, make sure to pinch off and completely close the fingers on the most distal aspect (*see figures 10-3 & 10-4*). This 'pinching off' is to be on the lateral and medial sides only so that the belly of the toenail is not engaged. Be careful at the pinch-off point that the client doesn't have a sharp or jagged toenail or you might get cut.

I am asked many times, "How many times do you twist on the way up?" from the hallux base. To answer this, you must have a good understanding of your client. If they're new you may only want to apply very gentle pressure and make two or three circular strides to the peak. As the client grows in appreciation for reflexology you may want to get their permission to use more pressure coupled with many more multiple twists to the peak.

I've done as many as twelve on my most experienced clients. That would give the average person so much pain, you would never see them again. So be very cautious with this important technique. Once you have worked this reflex move on to the hypothalamus to continue the dominant reflex hierarchy.

Hypothalamus – The Second Most Dominant Reflex

The hypothalamus is a small portion of the brain that is located below the thalamus just above the brain stem; it is roughly the size of an almond. One of the most important functions of the hypothalamus is to link the nervous system to the endocrine system via the pituitary gland.

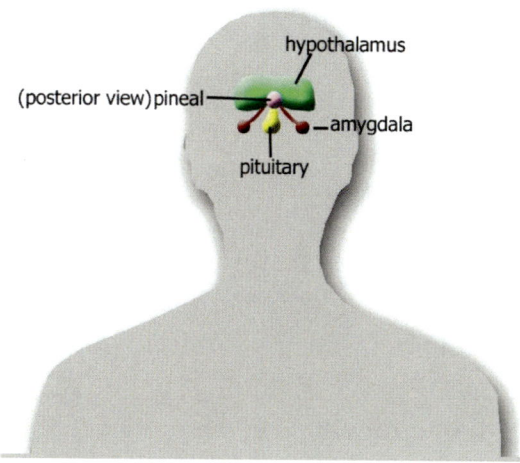

It synthesizes and secretes neurohormones, often called hypothalamic-releasing hormones, and these in turn stimulate or inhibit the secretion of pituitary hormones. These hormones affect gastric reflexes, hunger, blood pressure, feeding, anger, circadian cycles, maternal behavior, thirst, fatigue, immune responses, and control body temperature.

The pituitary is functionally linked to the hypothalamus by the pituitary stalk, whereby hypothalamic releasing factors are released and, in turn, stimulate the release of pituitary hormones. The *pituitary gland is known as the master endocrine gland.* But the *hypothalamus **truly** is the master over the endocrine system*, because it controls both lobes of the pituitary gland. Without the hypothalamus, life is not possible for humans. The hypothalamus, which is connected to the nervous system, also commands the pituitary for the benefit of our hormonal health. In other words, it unlocks the pituitary which balances and controls all hormones and their associated responsibilities.

The big reason I give, for the hypothalamus being the '**second most responsible reflex**' in unlocking the hierarchal reflex system is: The hypothalamus is responsible for the autonomic nervous system (sympathetic / parasympathetic nervous systems) as well as the hormonal system. It is this system that I am truly after for unlocking a way to the muscular and emotional blockages that are found in the body.

The hypothalamus must therefore respond to many different signals, some of which are generated externally and some internally but most noticeably from the central nervous system. This is why I believe in order for a patient to receive the benefits of reflexology, the central nervous system must be functioning properly. In Chapter Two, I mentioned my belief that paralyzed individuals cannot benefit from reflexology treatments. I base this observation by looking at the hypothalamus' role in the physiological system.

Chapter 10 – Hierarchal Treatment: The Dominant Reflexes

Pituitary / Pineal – The Third Most Dominant Reflex

The Pituitary Gland

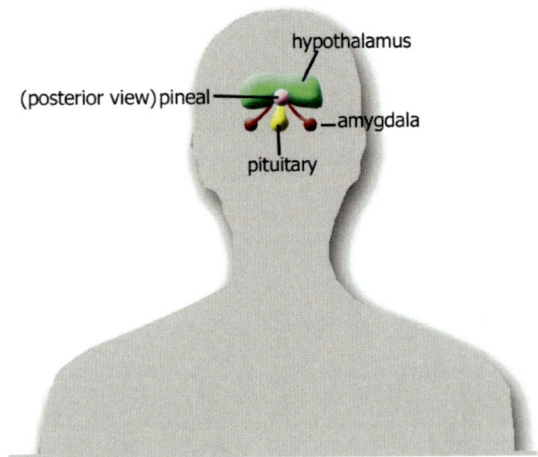

The pituitary gland is an endocrine gland that rests in a small, bony cavity off the bottom of the hypothalamus and is about the size of a pea.

The pituitary gland secretes hormones that stimulate other endocrine glands. It is widely known as the master gland of the body. It is functionally connected to the hypothalamus by the median eminence (which connects the hypothalamus with the anterior lobe of the pituitary gland).

The pituitary hormones have some dominion over the following body processes: Sex organ functions, aspects of pregnancy and childbirth, breast milk production, growth, thyroid gland function, blood pressure, metabolism, the Islets of Langerhans in the pancreas and water regulation in the body.

The pituitary gland is comprised of two lobes. The **Anterior Pituitary** and the **Posterior Pituitary** are separated by a thin layer of cells.

The Anterior Pituitary produces and secretes several important endocrine hormones: Growth hormone, beta endorphins, prolactin and thyroid-stimulating hormones among others.

The Posterior Pituitary secretes such hormones as oxytocin and vasopressin (ADH). Oxytocin stimulates uterine contractions and lactation. Vasopressin stimulates water retention, raises blood pressure by contracting arterioles and induces aggression in males.

A significant difference between the two lobes is that while the Posterior merely secretes hormones produced in the hypothalamus (to which it is attached), the Anterior pituitary produces AND secretes its hormones. Since this 'master gland' is under the control of the hypothalamus, I believe it's properly considered the third most dominant reflex along with the pineal gland. The two cannot be separated and if you are working one reflex you're working the other.

The Pineal Gland

The pineal gland is a very small organ, approximately one centimeter in size and shaped like a pine cone. It is attached to the posterior end of the roof of the third ventricle of the brain; anterior to the cerebellum; posterior to the hypothalamus and pituitary glands.

The gland's responsibility is to interpret the amount of light or the lack of it and determine how much melatonin to create and release. The secreting of melatonin is part of the parasympathetic response to the sympathetic adrenaline. Let me explain.

Adrenaline is released throughout the day to keep you awake and active. The pineal gland is stimulated by sunlight. However, we are creatures that require rest and sleep. So as the sun goes down, a hormone, in this case – melatonin – is triggered optically because of the lack of light.

What melatonin does is communicate with important endocrine glands to ease the adrenals to inhibit the secreting of adrenaline and cortisol. Breathing slows, muscles relax, the activity of the brain begins to wane; yawning, stretching and then sleep follows.

When the sun rises and the pineal deactivates the melatonin secretions and the sympathetic system begins to release adrenaline again (with the aid of cortisol for a short duration), the person wakes up to face another day.

However, when a person lives in a cloudy region or works a nighttime shift, the circadian cycle can be interrupted and make it difficult for the individual to sleep or stay awake. Many disorders can arise from the lack of sunlight. A person can overcome the night-shift induced sleep deprivation through training the circadian rhythms of the brain, but it seems preferable to use light for perfect sleep.

As the hypothalamus, pituitary and pineal glands are close in anatomical positioning I've put their reflex techniques under the same jurisdiction as seen on the next page.

Performing the Hypothalamus / Pituitary / Pineal Reflex Technique

The forefingers of the right hand should grip the back of the hallux, creating a vice-like grip. Without moving your fingers, swivel your elbow and wrist, swinging your hand above the foot being treated. It should feel like a key being turned 180° in the client's big toe (*see figures 10-5 & 10-6*). Once the hand is directly over the foot and the skin has been pulled taught – drive, then hook the thumb into the meaty tissue of the hallux pad.

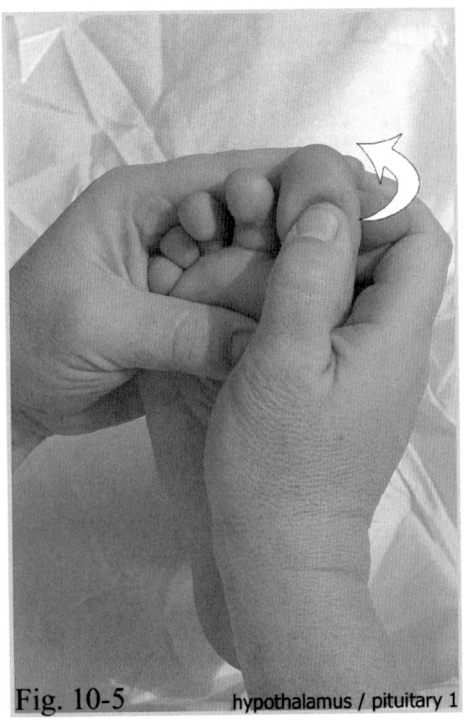

Fig. 10-5   hypothalamus / pituitary 1

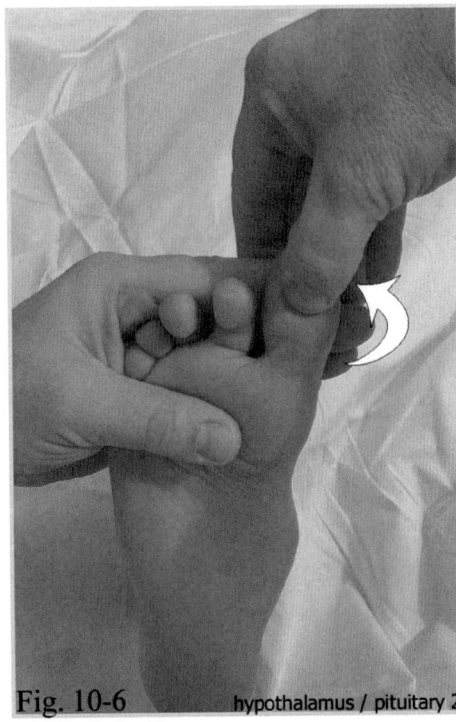

Fig. 10-6   hypothalamus / pituitary 2

With new clients, be careful of the amount of pressure applied to this reflex as it is a commonly sensitive area of the foot. This particular technique is to be used both on the hypothalamus and pituitary reflexes. What distinguishes the two separate reflexes is simply placing the thumb a little bit higher for the hypothalamus and a little bit lower for the pituitary. We're talking about less than 1/8 of an inch. As far as the hierarchal chart is concerned, we will use the technical terminology of the pituitary reflex lying in an inferior position to the hypothalamus. The hypothalamus and pituitary gland are so closely related that the reflex lies nearly in the same spot on the foot chart. If you strike one, you're pretty much striking the other at the same time. Therefore, the pituitary, which has 'Master' responsibilities becomes my third choice in the descending order that makes up the hierarchal reflexes.

Trapezius Shoulders – The Fourth Most Dominant Reflex

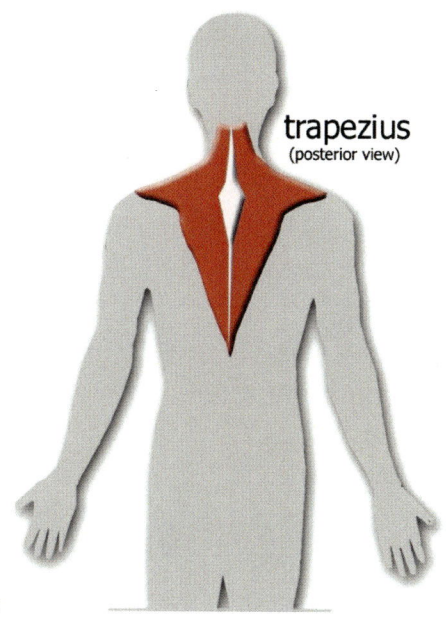

One great way to help the body to relax is when experienced hands squeeze the tired and tensed shoulders of a worn-out soul. Chair massages really sprang up in the 1990's because the focus in massage shifted. Clothes do not need to be shed; massages could be performed while the clients are still dressed. 'Who has time anymore? Great! Now I don't need to spend precious minutes taking my clothes off!'

However, this was a limited technique as most muscles could not be reached with the client still dressed. Since most people prefer that their shoulders and neck are rubbed first, it made sense for the commercial industry to capitalize on this market need. Thus, the advent of the massage chair – which appeared at every mall, sporting event and health club. What they were after were the large muscles that cover the entire shoulders, up the back of the neck, further still up to the back of the head.

The technical term for the shoulder muscles is the Trapezius. The trapezius is a large superficial muscle which extends longitudinally (or up and down) from the occipital bone (the back of the head) to the lower thoracic vertebrae (the mid- to low back), and laterally to the spine of the scapula (the shoulder blades).

The Trapezius gets its name from its trapezium-like shape when looking at both muscles at once: the corners being the neck, the two shoulders, and the thoracic vertebra (Thoracic 12). To me, it looks more like a kite.

An individual's behavior or mental state will determine how the shoulders will look or act under normal function. In other words, this 'state' is not during sports or the exaggerating of muscles during bodybuilding, rather just the general state of one's existence.

I'm going to describe how tension and stress can affect the way the trapezius muscles behave. It's important that we understand this, as reflexologists, because if we can get the shoulders to unlock – not only will it provide physical benefits of better circulation, it will also help to relax the whole body and improve the mental state of the individual.

To clarify: when a person gets a good chair massage on their shoulders, they walk away in a better condition. They will feel relaxed, be in a better mood and will feel 'good'. Yet, nothing in their life has changed from before they sat in that massage chair.

When someone has a lot of stress they tend to hold that stress in different areas of the anatomy. Women hold their stress in the hips, and most understand that the majority of men hold their stress in their shoulders and spine. I would hypothesize it resides in all three places, but in particular – the trapezius muscles.

Watch a particularly stressed client have the trapezius release while you're striking that reflex. It's an impressive thing to watch the shoulders widen as the neck elongates. How does this take place?

Scapular Elevation (the shrugging up or the lifting of the shoulders) occurs when the inferior fibers proceed upward and lateral-ward. Stress, over time, acts like a tourniquet. It pulls in and squeezes what should be loose, elongated muscles into short, tight, cramped muscles.

My observation over the years led me to recognize a unique way the body defends itself from stress. As the body defends itself from the worldly attacks on its association, it seems to retreat to a fetal position as a form of self-protection. My clients are unaware that this is even happening since it's on the subconscious level. You will see your clients 'sigh' and throw their shoulders back trying to release the stranglehold on their shoulders and self before a treatment.

What they're really doing is pulling their shoulder blades down in what we call **'scapular depression'** which is when the superior fibers of the trapezius are forced downward and laterally.

When that position does not feel comfortable, you will see the person throw their hands on the back of their head and force their elbows out and back as far as possible while leaning back into the chair. This may even happen during the treatment. This is referred to as **'scapular retraction'** (the drawing of the shoulder blades toward the midline) which is the forcing of the middle fibers to proceed horizontally and inwardly. Regardless of how the abnormalities came about or the ways the person tried to self-regulate the underlying issues, it is up to us as reflexologists to unlock this **fourth most dominant reflex**. I believe the unlocking of this reflex will make just as much of an impact on the emotional system as on the muscular system.

Performing the Trapezius Shoulders Reflex Technique

This technique is the most comprehensive one to learn. It involves a large area of the foot (both anterior and posterior aspects) as well as properly holding the foot while the working hand works in and around the digits (medially and laterally). It requires knowledge of when to work the reflexes up in a superior, longitudinal motion or when to simply work down the inferior aspects of the reflex area.

I do not I recommend working up the anterior trapezius on new clients. Start all techniques from the most distal aspects and work down on the digits. As they advance, move to the medial and lateral (interior) aspects of the digits. Save the superior maneuvers (upward motion to the distal part) for established clients because this is commonly a highly-sensitive directional reflex to work.

It amazes me that a client may feel less pain in the downward motion of the thumb-walking pressure but as soon as you change the direction and head back up the digits the pain can be excruciating.

Walking the Trapezius Ridge

I call this technique 'Walking the Ridge' because, as you can see in the image, the metatarsophalangeal joints protrude, creating a naturally-occurring ridge line for the thumb to walk across. Walking the trapezius ridge can be done from both directions; medial or lateral - it doesn't really matter which side you start. You will find, though that it is much more difficult to walk the ridge starting from the medial side. The reason for that is the crest of your hand between the thumb and index finger will come in contact with the hallux before the working thumb will make it to the 5th metatarsal head.

Those of us with bigger hands have it a little easier. If you have small hands you will have to release your forefingers of the working hand from the dorsal aspect of the foot and let them slide over the top of the toes to reach the last position. From the lateral side you should be able to reach all positions of the ridge.

Chapter 10 – Hierarchal Treatment: The Dominant Reflexes

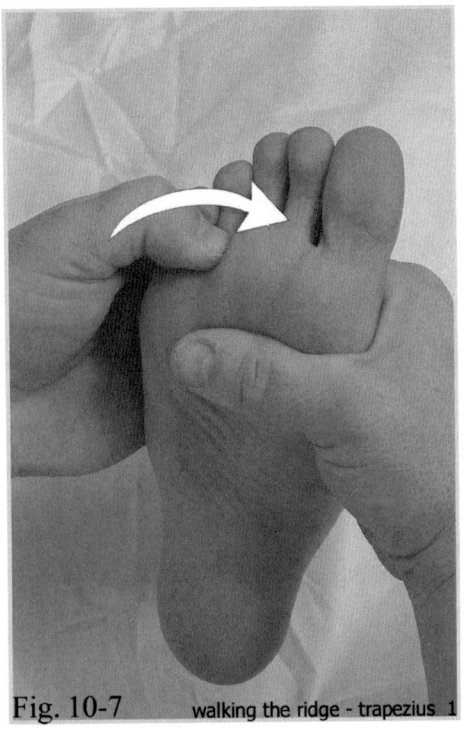

Fig. 10-7   walking the ridge - trapezius 1

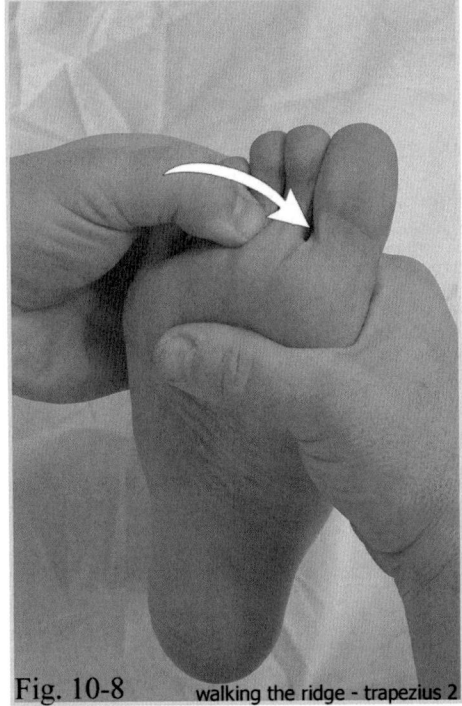

Fig. 10-8   walking the ridge - trapezius 2

Start by placing the holding hand with the thumb just below the metatarsal heads while the forefingers lie on the dorsal aspect from the medial side. Keep a firm hold as you take your working hand and laterally position it over the 5th metatarsal head at the metatarsophalangeal joint (*see figure 10-7*).

The working hand fingers should rest gently on the dorsal aspect of the foot just over the working fingers of your working hand. In other words, your holding hand should be in contact with the epidermis on the dorsal aspect and your working hand should be folded over your holding hand and not touching the foot's epidermis at all.

Begin striking the most lateral aspect of the foot by deeply penetrating the dermis and soft tissue. Allow your thumb to feel the deep grooves between the joints as you walk the entire ridge (*see figure 10-8*). Make sure not to skip the soft areas between the bony protrusions. Work all the way to the most medial aspect below the hallux base.

Chapter 10 – Hierarchal Treatment: The Dominant Reflexes

Plantar Digits Down (Anterior Trapezius)

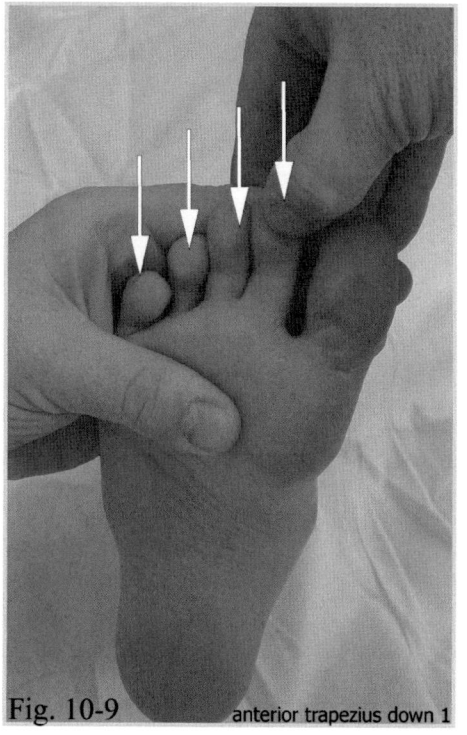
Fig. 10-9   anterior trapezius down 1

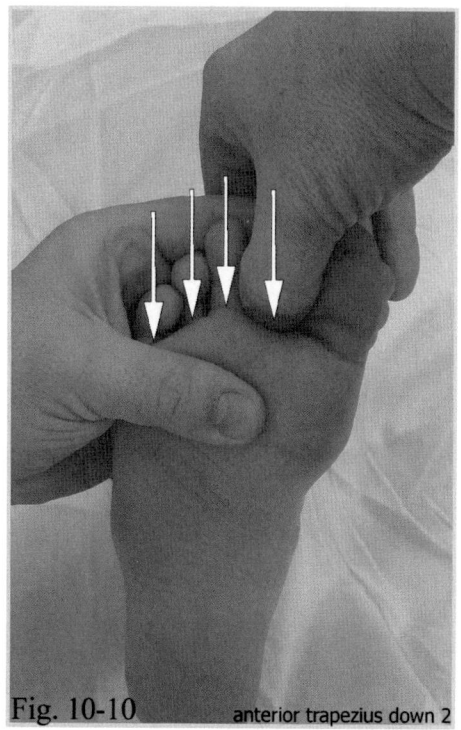
Fig. 10-10   anterior trapezius down 2

Reverse the holding hand to the lateral side of the foot. Make sure the index finger of the holding hand holds the transverse plain of the dorsal aspect of the foots phalanges. The thumb of the working hand should hold firm to the plantar transverse plain.

Use the thumb of the working hand to inch its way down the plantar surface of the toes (from distal to proximal) until you reach the digit's greatest depth (*see figures 10-9 & and 10-10*). The more advanced your client becomes you may work the medial and lateral sides of the toes from the top to bottom.

Plantar Digits Up (Anterior Trapezius)

This reflex technique is reserved for advanced clients whose pain tolerance has increased with each treatment and have the understanding that pain from reflexology is a benefit. Use the same holding technique as you would with Plantar Digits Down (anterior trapezius). With the

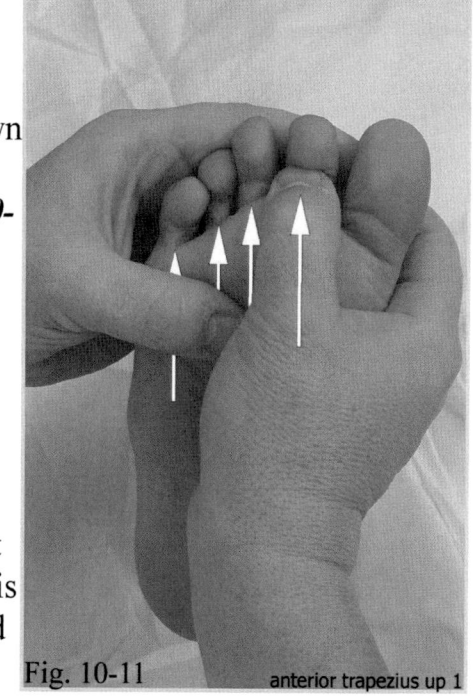
Fig. 10-11   anterior trapezius up 1

114

thumb of the working hand begin at the base of the phalanges and work up (in a superior longitudinal direction) to the top of the digit (*see figure 10-11*). Drive as much blood as possible to the tip of the toe. Make sure that the fingers of the working hand overlap the fingers of the holding hand while the thumb of the working hand drives upward on each digit.

When working the toes, stop at the crest of the toe making sure not to hit the nail. Remember, this can be very painful to new clients so discretion is needed on the part of the practitioner.

Dorsal Digits Down (Posterior Trapezius)

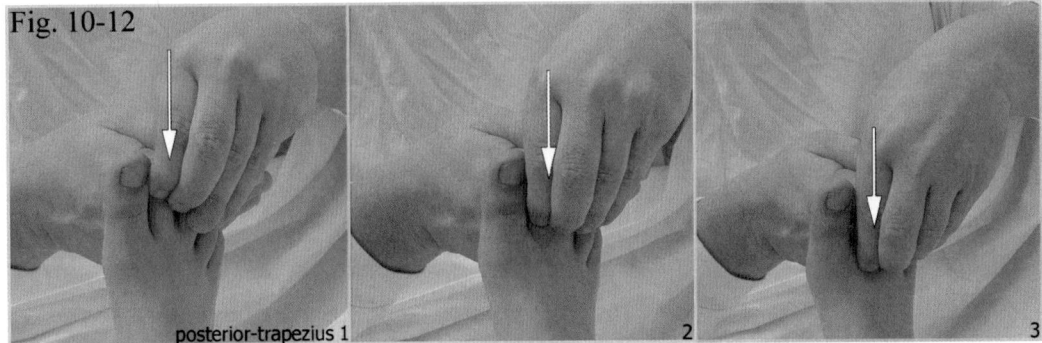

You may use one or all of your working hand fingers to strike the posterior reflex of the trapezius. I tend to mix and match the fingers used depending on the condition of the toes. Are they hammered or bent in unusual directions? The answer will affect leverage of both the holding hand and the working hand when reaching these reflexes.

Lay the dorsal part of your holding hand against the plantar aspect of the foot across the transverse plain. Open the working hand, stretching the forefingers up and over the distal part of the toes, sliding the thumb between the thumb of the holing hand and its fingers (*see figure 10-12*). By pinching the thumb of the working hand with the thumb and fingers of the holding hand will help you gain leverage for striking the dorsal aspect of the foot's digits.

Hip Sciatic – The Fifth Most Dominant Reflex

The sciatic nerve is a large nerve that starts in the lower back and runs through the buttock and down the leg to the feet. It is the **longest and widest single nerve** in the body, measuring about three-quarters of an inch in diameter. It supplies the skin of the leg, the back thigh muscles as well as those of the leg and foot. The sciatic nerve enables motor and sensory functions (movement and feeling) in the thigh, knee, calf, ankle, **foot and toes**. Originating in the sacral plexus (a network of nerves that serves the pelvis, buttocks, genitals, thighs, calves, and feet) located in the low back – the nerve enters the lower limb (the leg) by exiting the pelvis through the greater sciatic foramen (the opening in the pelvic bone).

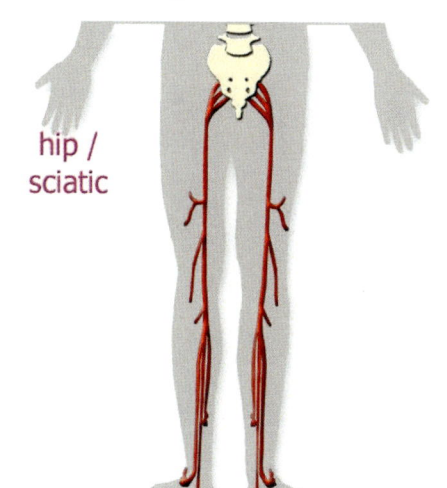

One of the biggest problems we see as reflexologists is sciatica. **Sciatica** is a problem where pain is caused by a compression or irritation of the sciatic nerve by an issue in the lower back. Degenerative disk disease and spinal stenosis are some of the low-back conditions that could cause sciatica. This is not to be confused with the SI joint which can simulate sciatica.

The **sacroiliac joint** or SI joint is the joint between the sacrum, at the base of the spine and the ilium of the pelvis, which are joined by ligaments. It is a strong, weight-bearing synovial joint with irregular elevations and depressions that produce interlocking of the two bones.

The human body has two sacroiliac joints - a left and a right joint. The sacroiliac joints are located at the bottom of the back. You have one on either side of the spine. The sacroiliac joints help make up the rear part of the pelvic girdle and sit between the sacrum and the ilia. Inflammation of these joints can radiate pain down the leg just like sciatica. But remember, one is from issues from the spine while the other is an issue related to the hip joint. It is interesting, however, that working the low back sciatic reflexes help both conditions at the same time. It's as if you are killing two birds with one stone.

I have also found that weak muscles of the core contribute to this problem because the lower posture of the lumbars is not suspended with strong muscles of the low back.

There is something else that I feel may be profound when sciatica develops. I believe women in particular also hold stress in the low back, as well as the shoulders. If I had to pick one over the other, I would work the shoulders because it unlocks the upper torso and muscular system. But the low back is very important because it unlocks emotional issues as well as nerve innervation for the whole spine. The proof has been in the field. How so?

Even after a client has received many SI and lumbar adjustments from their chiropractor to try and treat chronic sciatica, the condition may continue. There really is no reason for the nerve to keep referring pain to the individual because the facets are open and freely suspending. Well, that is…if we look at it from an allopathic point of view only.

From the holistic side, the root cause may not always be deemed **clinical**. This is not to be viewed as mystic, rather an unorthodox attempt at finding new truths by looking at the entire nature of man. What am I getting at?

There is no doubt in my mind that **nerves** are affected by stress. Stress interferes with biochemical reactions as well as electrochemical pulses needed for daily diagnosis of one self. Sciatic pain can arise from stressed nerves or the compression (cutting off) of healthy pulses, causing the brain to misdiagnose issues.

The women I have been privileged to work on over the years have told me how much better they feel after we unlock the hip / sciatic reflex. Some women cry, some glow, and others just sigh as the stress is thrown from the body from the engaging of this painful reflex. On their return visits they inform me that they no longer suffer radiating pain down the leg nor the symptoms of **restless leg** syndrome.

Men, too, have been known to hold stress in the low back, but my experience shows their low back pain to be more clinical.

Working the sciatic reflex thoroughly will unlock the hips and low back, allowing for premium spinal nerve innervation to succeed. This is why I made the hip / sciatic reflex the **5th most dominant** reflex to be worked.

Chapter 10 – Hierarchal Treatment: The Dominant Reflexes

Performing the Hip Sciatic Reflex

This is one reflex area that allows for a lot of freedom when executing these reflex techniques. You may use one, two, three or all fingers to reach multiple reflexes. Acceptable forms would include hooking, digging, driving, torque and press, rocking, and extension with compression to meet the needs of the client.

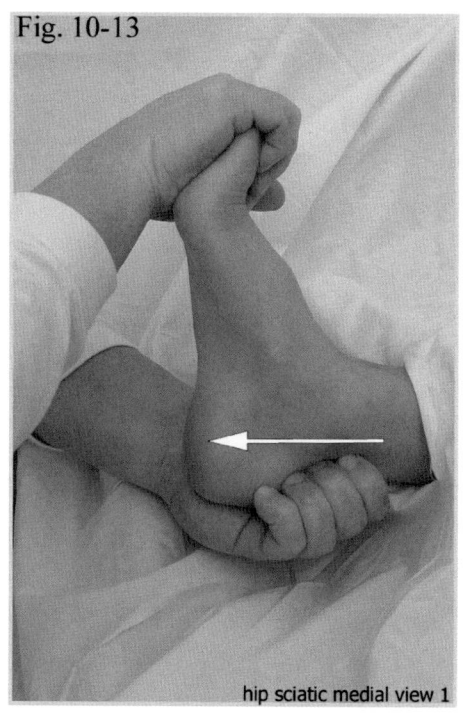

Fig. 10-13

This is where your personal art can shine. However, here are some basics I have developed over the years that can act as a launching point in your career. Use them as the foundation to your approach to the hip / sciatic reflex.

In *figure 10-13*, you can see the palm of the working hand is on the lateral aspect of the ankle while the forefingers are squeezing the medial side. Squeeze (compression) then release (relax your fingers) as you pull back on the foot with the working hand.

Use the holding hand to stabilize the transverse plane using the palm of the holding hand against the plantar aspect. Start at the notch in the skin just under the talus bone and work towards the heel of the foot. Make sure to work all posterior aspects not missing any part of the planar surface. We'll call this exercise '**medial compression and extension of the hip / sciatic**'.

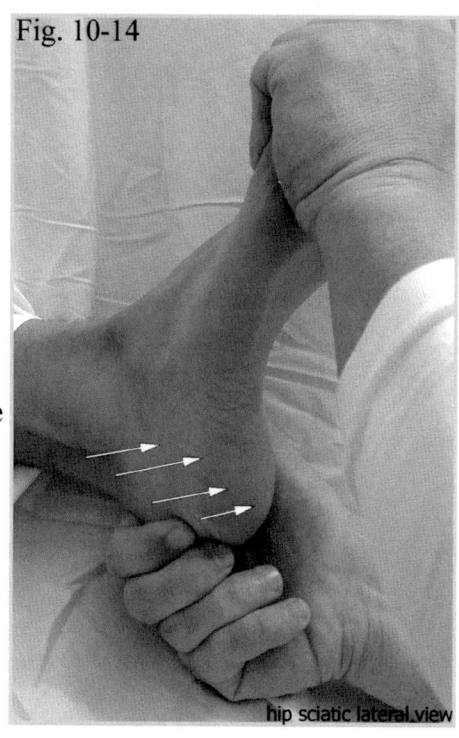

Fig. 10-14

In *figure 10-14*, just reverse the process. We will call that exercise '**lateral compression and extension of the hip / sciatic**'.

Chapter 10 – Hierarchal Treatment: The Dominant Reflexes

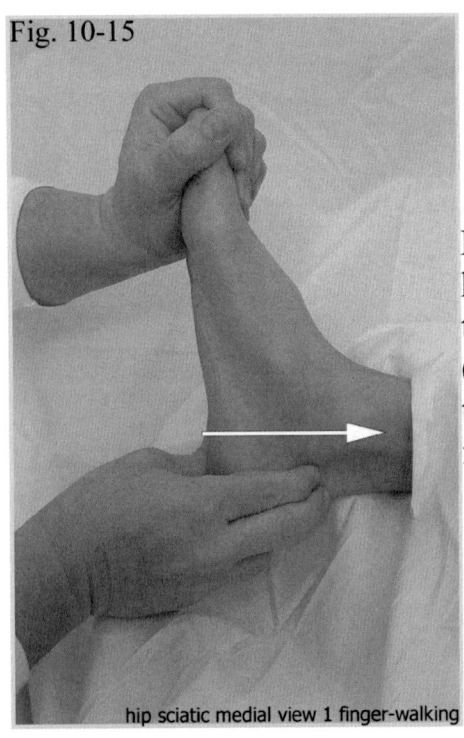
hip sciatic medial view 1 finger-walking

In *figure 10-15*, use the first few digits of the working hand to work inferior to superior on the medial aspect of the hip / sciatic reflex using forward finger drive (acupressure). Again, use the holding hand to stabilize transverse plane. We will call this exercise **'medial finger drive of the hip / sciatic'**.

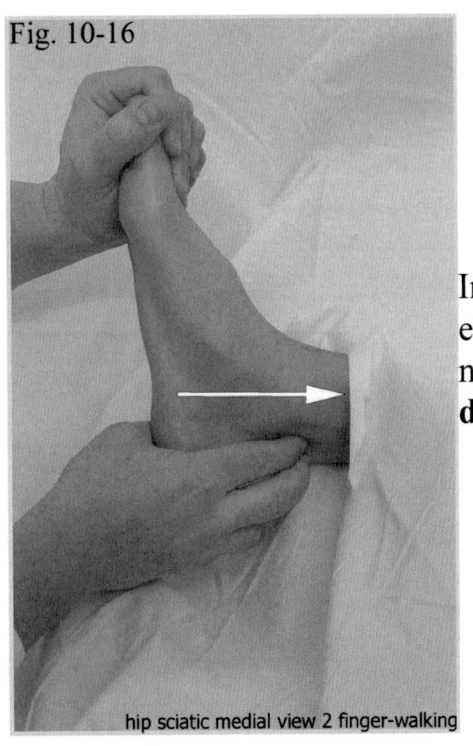
hip sciatic medial view 2 finger-walking

In *figure 10-16*, simply reverse the process. You can even lower the holding hand for more leverage if needed. This exercise will be called **'lateral finger drive of the hip / sciatic'**.

Chapter 10 – Hierarchal Treatment: The Dominant Reflexes

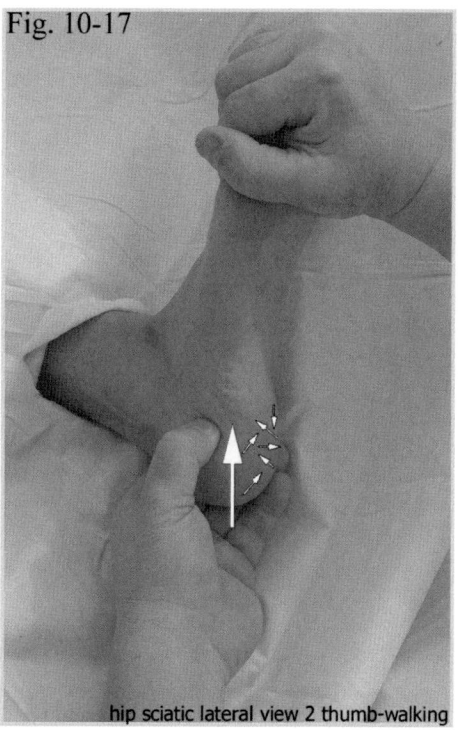

Fig. 10-17

hip sciatic lateral view 2 thumb-walking

In *figure 10-17*, use your thumb of the working hand to drive deep in the dermis of the entire heel pad (plantar pad). You have to switch hands often. There is an infinite number of ways to drive, hook and compress the fingers to reach these low back reflexes. So do not limit yourself to my basic techniques. Work in as many directions as possible. I can't stress enough the need to strike every part of the heel and adjoining structures.

Spine – The Sixth and Last of the Dominant Reflexes

The spine (also known as the backbone) is a vertebral column comprised of **26 vertebrae**. It is located in the dorsal aspect of the torso. Each vertebra is separated by spinal discs and in its spinal canal it housed the spinal cord.

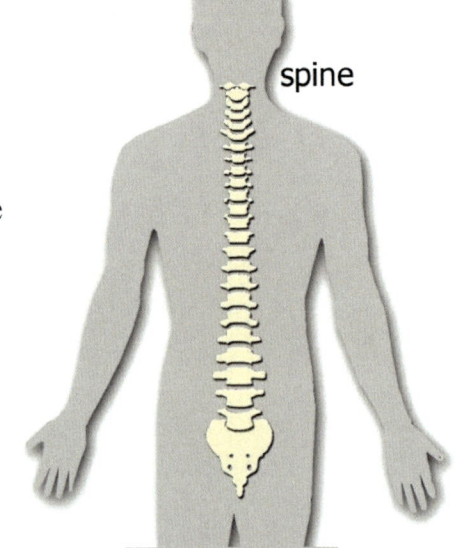

The spine presents several curves when viewed laterally and these curves delineate the different regions: the **cervicals (7)**, the **thoracics (12)**, the **lumbars (5)** and the **sacral/coccyx (2)**.

Convexing forward, the **cervical curve** begins at the apex of the odontoid (or tooth-like) process and ends at the middle of the second thoracic vertebra. It is the least marked of all the curves; comprised of the smallest-bodied vertebra.

Concaving forward and known as a *tt curve,* the **thoracic curve** begins at the middle of the second thoracic vertebrae and ends at the middle of the twelfth thoracic.
The **lumbar curve**, also known as a *lordotic curve*, begins at the middle of the last thoracic vertebra, and ends at the sacrovertebral angle. It convexes anteriorly and this curve is more marked in females than in males. The pelvic curve begins at the sacrovertebral articulation and ends at the coccyx while concaving directionally downward and forward.

The vertebrae are divided into five parts listed here superior to inferior:

1. Cervicals – C1 through C7. C1 is known as the "atlas' while C2 is the axis.
2. Thoracics – T1 through T12. These possess costal facets for articulating the heads of the ribs.
3. Lumbars – L1 through L5. They are larger but lack the costal facets of the thoracics.
4. Sacral region – S1 through S5. The vertebrae in the sacral region are fused. I found out the reason for the five bones fusing later on in a child's life after having kids of my own. Have you ever watched a small child bounce on their butt as they play on the kitchen floor? If those bones were not soft and unjoined they would make the perfect spear that would puncture the lower region of the small intestine

or colon. I guess that's why we, as adults, don't bounce on our backside, because of the now-fused sacral bones.
5. Coccygeal – also called the tailbone. It is comprised of three-to-five fused vertebrae.

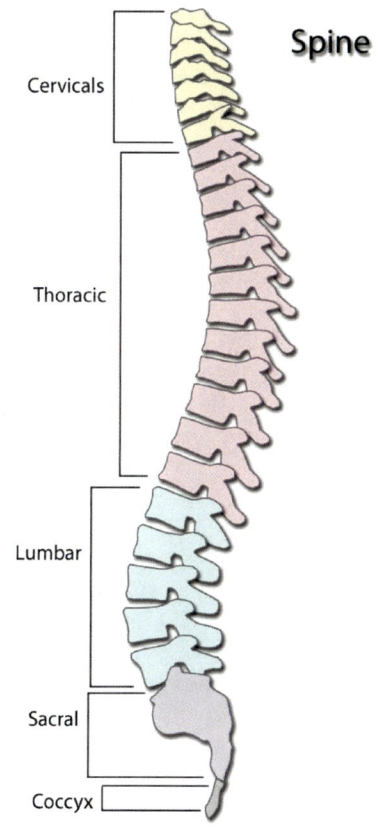

Some people have abnormal curvatures of the spine. The most common of them is Scoliosis, a lateral curvature, and more common among females and may result from unequal growth of the two sides of one or more vertebrae or asymmetrical musculature on one side of the spine. Other symptoms are: Unequal distance between the body and arms, in females – asymmetric size or location of breasts, differing shoulder heights as well as hip and rib cage levels and finally, slow nerve action (although this is not in all cases).

A couple of other slightly less common conditions: often seen in osteoporosis is the "dowager's hump", also called kyphosis; where it presents itself as an exaggerated posterior curvature in the thoracic region of the spine. Another is Lordosis (and seen in pregnant women is called Temporary Lordosis); where there is an exaggerated anterior curvature in the lumbar region.

The **vertebral canal**, which houses the spinal cord, follows the different curves of the column. In the parts of the spinal column that have the greatest mobility, like the cervicals and lumbars, it is large and triangularly-shaped. In the thoracic region, where mobility is more limited, it is small and rounded.

The central nervous system is composed of the brain and spinal cord. The brain has **12 cranial nerves** (5 motor nerves, 3 sensory nerves, 4 nerves motor/sensory) and **31 pairs of spinal nerves** (8 pair cervical, 12 pair thoracic, 5 pair lumbar, 5 pair sacral, 1 pair coccyx). The spinal cord provides means of communication between the brain and **peripheral nerves**. It is this system that we, as reflexologists, must have intact to achieve our objective. This system is so complex that very little is truly known how it works. But we do have this basic information that guides us in understanding how reflexology might work.

Chapter 10 – Hierarchal Treatment: The Dominant Reflexes

Some basic diseases that can be spine-related:

- Chronic back pain
- Degenerative Disc Disease
- Endometriosis
- Foot pain related to back pain and lumbar injury
- Fibromyalgia
- Kidney Stone
- Osteoporosis
- Sciatica
- Spina Bifida

- A discussion of spinal abnormalities will continue but a chart that gives insight to the nerve innervation of the spine is included on the following page.

Chapter 10 – Hierarchal Treatment: The Dominant Reflexes

Effects of Spinal Misalignments

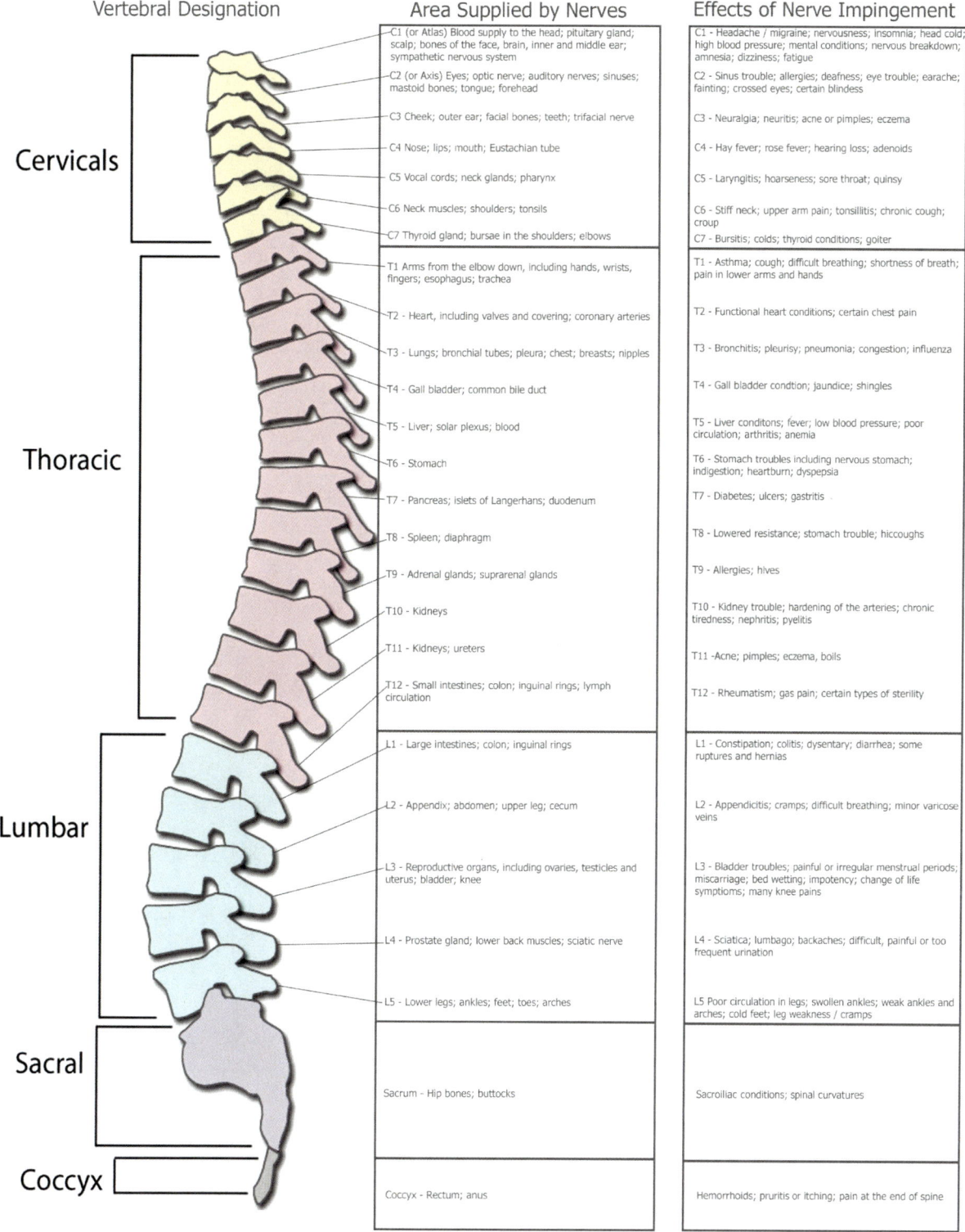

Vertebral Designation	Area Supplied by Nerves	Effects of Nerve Impingement
Cervicals	C1 (or Atlas) Blood supply to the head; pituitary gland; scalp; bones of the face, brain, inner and middle ear; sympathetic nervous system	C1 - Headache / migraine; nervousness; insomnia; head cold; high blood pressure; mental conditions; nervous breakdown; amnesia; dizziness; fatigue
	C2 (or Axis) Eyes; optic nerve; auditory nerves; sinuses; mastoid bones; tongue; forehead	C2 - Sinus trouble; allergies; deafness; eye trouble; earache; fainting; crossed eyes; certain blindess
	C3 Cheek; outer ear; facial bones; teeth; trifacial nerve	C3 - Neuralgia; neuritis; acne or pimples; eczema
	C4 Nose; lips; mouth; Eustachian tube	C4 - Hay fever; rose fever; hearing loss; adenoids
	C5 Vocal cords; neck glands; pharynx	C5 - Laryngitis; hoarseness; sore throat; quinsy
	C6 Neck muscles; shoulders; tonsils	C6 - Stiff neck; upper arm pain; tonsillitis; chronic cough; croup
	C7 Thyroid gland; bursae in the shoulders; elbows	C7 - Bursitis; colds; thyroid conditions; goiter
Thoracic	T1 Arms from the elbow down, including hands, wrists, fingers; esophagus; trachea	T1 - Asthma; cough; difficult breathing; shortness of breath; pain in lower arms and hands
	T2 - Heart, including valves and covering; coronary arteries	T2 - Functional heart conditions; certain chest pain
	T3 - Lungs; bronchial tubes; pleura; chest; breasts; nipples	T3 - Bronchitis; pleurisy; pneumonia; congestion; influenza
	T4 - Gall bladder; common bile duct	T4 - Gall bladder condtion; jaundice; shingles
	T5 - Liver; solar plexus; blood	T5 - Liver conditons; fever; low blood pressure; poor circulation; arthritis; anemia
	T6 - Stomach	T6 - Stomach troubles including nervous stomach; indigestion; heartburn; dyspepsia
	T7 - Pancreas; islets of Langerhans; duodenum	T7 - Diabetes; ulcers; gastritis
	T8 - Spleen; diaphragm	T8 - Lowered resistance; stomach trouble; hiccoughs
	T9 - Adrenal glands; suprarenal glands	T9 - Allergies; hives
	T10 - Kidneys	T10 - Kidney trouble; hardening of the arteries; chronic tiredness; nephritis; pyelitis
	T11 - Kidneys; ureters	T11 - Acne; pimples; eczema, boils
	T12 - Small intestines; colon; inguinal rings; lymph circulation	T12 - Rheumatism; gas pain; certain types of sterility
Lumbar	L1 - Large intestines; colon; inguinal rings	L1 - Constipation; colitis; dysentary; diarrhea; some ruptures and hernias
	L2 - Appendix; abdomen; upper leg; cecum	L2 - Appendicitis; cramps; difficult breathing; minor varicose veins
	L3 - Reproductive organs, including ovaries, testicles and uterus; bladder; knee	L3 - Bladder troubles; painful or irregular menstrual periods; miscarriage; bed wetting; impotency; change of life symptoms; many knee pains
	L4 - Prostate gland; lower back muscles; sciatic nerve	L4 - Sciatica; lumbago; backaches; difficult, painful or too frequent urination
	L5 - Lower legs; ankles; feet; toes; arches	L5 Poor circulation in legs; swollen ankles; weak ankles and arches; cold feet; leg weakness / cramps
Sacral	Sacrum - Hip bones; buttocks	Sacroiliac conditions; spinal curvatures
Coccyx	Coccyx - Rectum; anus	Hemorrhoids; pruritis or itching; pain at the end of spine

Chapter 10 – Hierarchal Treatment: The Dominant Reflexes

The spine must be unlocked to allow for the preservation of nerve innervation for it, as well as its adjoining members. It allows for nerve supply needed in the brain's ability for self diagnostics as well as stimulating relaxation to the entire nervous system. It is our key to make the brain work for us through the initiation of reflexes. It is this system that replies to us what goes on in the internal system. And it is this structure that allows us to heal the body from within.

Therefore the spine reflex is the final member **(6) on the most dominant list**.

Performing the Spine Reflex

To work the cervicals, use the holding hand to grip the toes as well as part of the transverse area over the 5th metatarsal head (*see figure 10-18*). Keep a firm hold on the toes without pinching the dorsal side of the foot. Open up the working hand and use gentle leverage with the thumb on the plantar aspect and the forefingers on the dorsal side.

Use the index finger to drive up the cervical reflex. You can also work **anteroposterior** (front to back). The cervicals start right around the metatarso-interphalangeal joint (clavicle guideline) of the hallux and end just before the crown of the big toe. To strike the thoracic reflexes, simply move the working hand down the mid foot and switch from using the index finger to using the thumb (*see figure 10-19*).

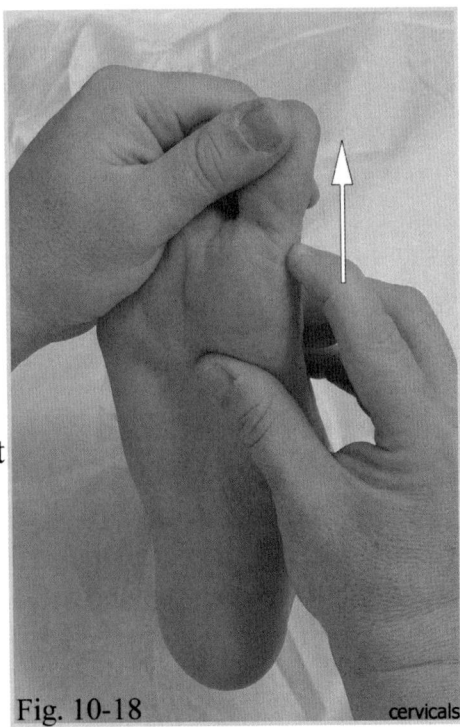

Fig. 10-18   cervicals

As the thumb drives, make sure to slid the forefingers across the dorsal aspect. Let them remain in firm contact with the skin. They will be your counter-lever to the thumb's downward pressure. The thoracic reflexes start around the cuboid-transverse guideline and end at the clavicle guideline. The lumbar reflexes start around the plantar pad, where the soft skin becomes thick and runs along the medial plain up to the cuboid transverse guideline. The sacral-coccyx spinal reflexes lie about a half-inch below the start of the lumbars.

If I ask my students to strike the sacral reflex during the practical exam and they are

Chapter 10 – Hierarchal Treatment: The Dominant Reflexes

below the cuboid-transverse line but above the plantar pad transition, they will have missed the mark. Remember, the last two bones will be just below the beginning of the lumbar reflex which puts you inferior to the plantar pad guideline.

Reserved for the more experienced client is the spinal reflex technique on *figures 10-20 & 10-21*.

This technique will be surprisingly painful as you use the two digits of the working hand to drive the medial flesh transecting the longitudinal axis. When moving inferior to superior up the foot, work all the way from the plantar surface to the dorsal side.

Exaggerate the movement beyond the spinal chart's guidelines; that way you make sure to strike every aspect of the spine. You will find that your index finger will do more work than your second digit. That's okay, but if the index is tired, simply lift the index finger and allow the second digit to work harder.

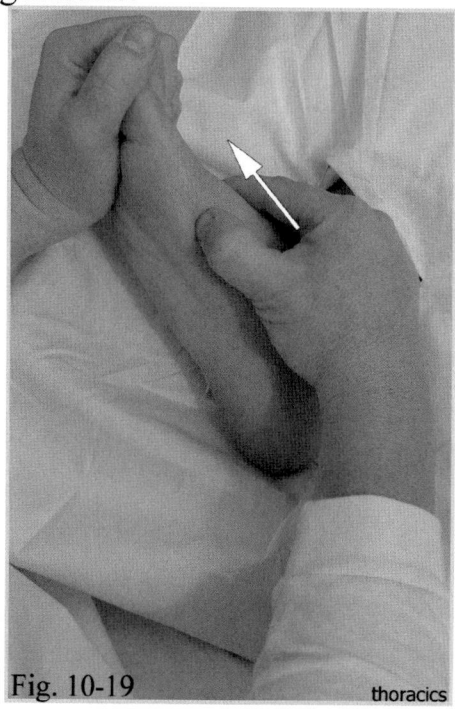

Fig. 10-19 — thoracics

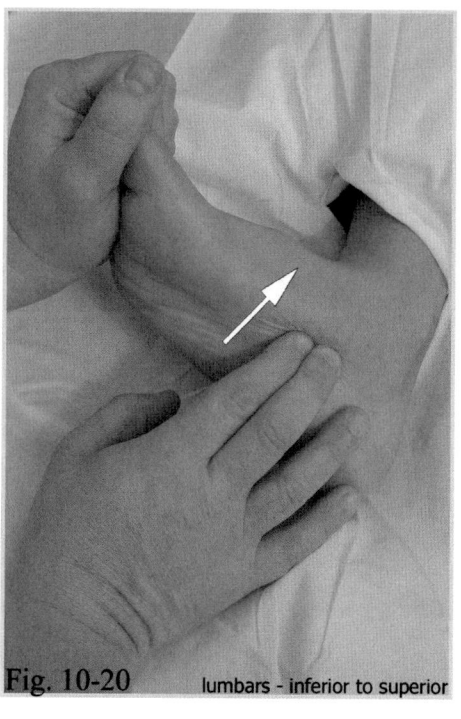

Fig. 10-20 — lumbars - inferior to superior

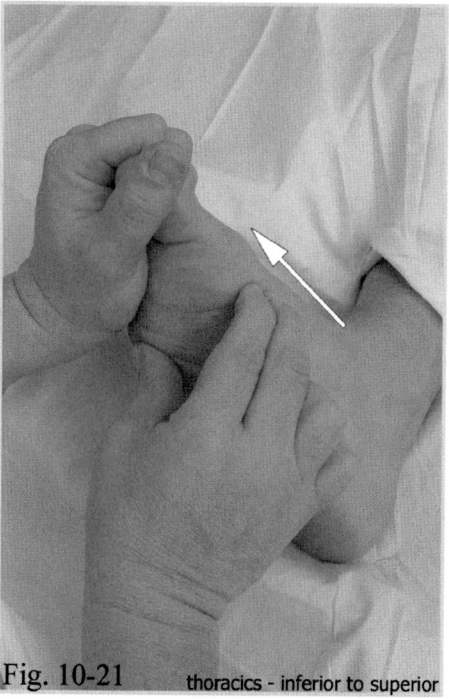

Fig. 10-21 — thoracics - inferior to superior

Chapter 10 – Hierarchal Treatment: The Dominant Reflexes

****

All in all, the dominant reflexes open the way for intermedial reflexes to be stimulated and determine who is in charge of the health exercise. The reflexologist gains control of the client's system and overrides the nervous system to achieve his goals.

Chapter 10 – Hierarchal Treatment: The Dominant Reflexes

Chapter Eleven

Hierarchal Treatment:

The Intermedial Reflexes

Hierarchal Treatment – Intermedial Reflexes

In this chapter we will discuss how to perform the Intermedial reflex techniques and an explanation as to how these reflexes affect the hierarchy and value to the entire physiological association.

Occipitalis – The Alpha of the Intermedial Reflexes

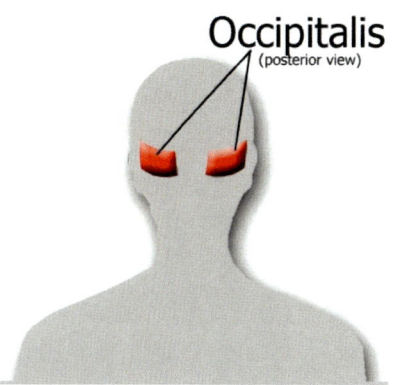

The **Occipitalis** (**ox**-sip-ih-**tay**-lis) Muscle lies on the posterior side of the head over the occipital bone and attaches to the **Frontalis** (frun-**tay**-lis) Muscle which lies over the frontal bone over the anterior aspect of the head. These two muscles, along with the tendinous membrane that attaches them – referred to as the **Galea** (**gay**-lee-uh), are called the **Epicranius Muscle** covering the cranium like a cap.

The occipitalis muscles do not extend fully across the back of the head as they are connected in the middle by the galea. Contraction of these muscles raises the eyebrows and causes the forehead skin to wrinkle horizontally. Continued contraction of these muscles (due to stress and anxiety) are known to cause tension headaches.

A constant theme of stress is watching men and women rub the front, back and sides of their head to relieve pain from a tension headache. This tension and stress, I believe, stems from the trapezius muscles (from consistent scapular elevation) and works its way up the back of the head to the occipitalis. This reflex when worked properly should bring relief to not only the facial muscles of the forehead but also relieve tension and stress to the back of the head helping to relieve the common headache.

When a client with this type of headache sits in front of me, this particular reflex will be sensitive and working it will sometimes bring them instant relief. Regardless, I believe this reflex opens circulation to the occipital nerves, which would unlock and open the necessary nerve response for relief to the occipital region.

Chapter 11 – Hierarchal Treatment: Intermedial Reflexes

Performing the Occipitalis Reflexes

Notice how the holding hand grabs hold of the toes in *figure 11-1*. See how the index finger of the holding hand is just on the tip of the nail while the thumb is pinching ever so lightly the plantar part of the hallux. The thumb gives leverage that will counteract the pressure of the working hand.

While using the thumb of the working hand to hold the interphalangeal joint of the hallux steady, use the index finger to 'inch' its way from the spinal reflex's longitudinal line all the way around to the lateral aspect of the hallux's longitudinal line. Your finger will work the slight curve of the dorsal aspect of the toe similar to a half-moon.

Get as close to the nail bed as possible, even touching the nail itself on the dorsal aspect and work your way down to the base of the hallux. This reflex can be quite sensitive to first-time reflexology clients so be careful.

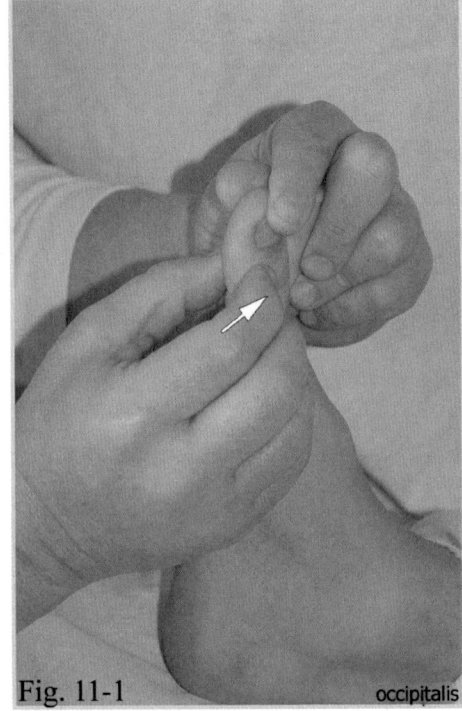

Fig. 11-1   occipitalis

Sternocleidomastoid / Neck – the Second of the Intermedial Reflexes

In human anatomy, the sternocleidomastoid (**stir**-no-**kly**-doh-mass-toyd) muscle is a paired muscle in the superficial layers of the anterior portion of the neck. It acts to flex and rotate the head.

It is called such because it originates at the uppermost segment of the sternum (sterno-) and the clavicle (cleido-), and has an insertion at the mastoid process (inferior posterior) of the temporal bone of the skull.

This muscle passes obliquely across the side of the neck. The sternocleidomastoid is within the investing fascia of the neck, along with the trapezius muscle, with which it shares its nerve supply (the accessory nerve).

Many important structures relate to the sternocleidomastoid, including the common **carotid** (kuh-**raw**-tid) artery (main blood supply to the brain), accessory nerve (nerve supply also to the trapezius muscles), and brachial (**bray**-kee-ul) **plexus** (a network of nerves that is formed by the lower four cervical nerves and the first thoracic nerve supplying nerves to the chest, shoulder, and arm).

Even though I believe that the trapezius muscle is the most dominant reflex for unlocking the muscular system it is prudent to identify the importance of the sternocleidomastoid and how it can cut off nerve supply to the trapezius; so it does have importance in the overall release of the muscular system.

Performing the Sternocleidomastoid / Neck Reflexes

See the holding hand in *figure 11-2* as it, like in the occipitalis, takes hold of all the toes. The index finger of the holding hand is below the nail while the thumb is lightly pinching the plantar part of the hallux at its distal aspect.

The index finger of both the holding hand and the working hand provide leverage against the thumb of the working hand which drives across the head of the metatarso-interphalangeal joint and works obliquely to the lateral aspect of the side-of-neck reflex.

Chapter 11 – Hierarchal Treatment: Intermedial Reflexes

Make several passes medial to lateral to effectively strike this reflex. As your client progresses in pain tolerance and homeostasis, rotate the toe with the holding hand abductionally as you thumb-drive. This will increase the intensity of the sternocleidomastoid reflex.

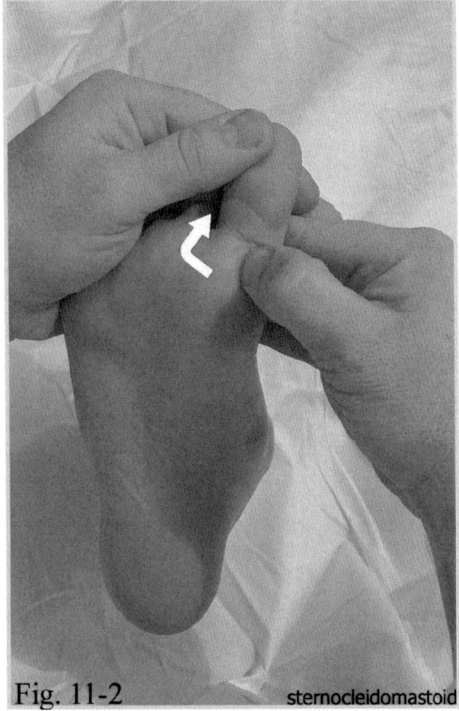

Fig. 11-2   sternocleidomastoid

Thyroid / Parathyroid - the Third of the Intermedial Reflexes

The **Thyroid** is one of the largest endocrine glands in the body and is controlled by the hypothalamus and pituitary.

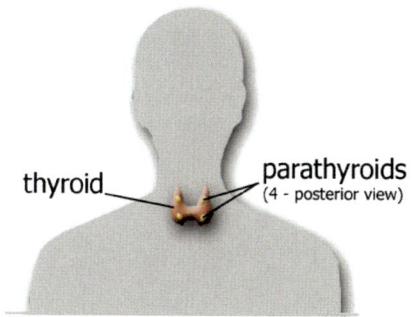

This gland is found in the neck inferior to the thyroid cartilage (Adam's apple). It is composed of two cone-like lobes or wings resembling a butterfly in flight.

The thyroid controls how quickly the body burns energy, makes proteins, and how sensitive the body should be to other hormones. It has a strong influence over the testes and the ovaries as well as the adrenal glands. The thyroid also produces the hormone **calcitonin**, which contributes to the regulation of blood calcium levels in the body.

Thyroid hormones regulate the rate of metabolism (hypo or hyper) and affect the growth and rate of function of many other systems in the body.

Women ask me all the time if working the thyroid can lead to weight loss. I wish it was that simple. However, hypothyroidism is the enemy of everyone who want to keep the weight off.

Two common thyroid issues we want to get familiar with:

Hyperthyroidism (overactive thyroid). When this issue arises we will see significant weight loss, vomiting, increased blood pressure, or a persistently fast heart rate. Some feel they are bouncing off walls (nervousness) and sweating all the time.

Hyperthyroidism also effects the skin in many ways:
- Thickening of the epidermis
- Fast nail growth
- Rough, dry skin
- Increased pigmentation
- Increased skin temperature
- Red palms
- Increased sweating palms, soles

Hypothyroidism (underactive thyroid). When we see issues such as fatigue, poor attention, weight gain, numbness, and tingling of the hands or feet, we would generally blame this state on the hypo-side. Changes to the skin are not limited to hyperthyroidism. Hypothyroidism can even have a greater impact on our skin. Women complain to me all the time about these conditions (which also effect men):

- Pale, cold, scaly, wrinkled skin
- Coarse, dry scalp and hair
- Cannot Sweat
- Hair loss
- Yellowish skin color
- Edema (puffy hands, face, eyelids)
- Thick brittle nails
- Eczema
- Bruises easily

Thyroid can make a difference on how cold we feel which is the top complaint of women over 60 in my practice. Some of my clients reported that with each year they age their body feels colder and colder.

The life of the thyroid is Iodine. It is the food that makes homeostasis of this endocrine gland possible. As diet continues to degrade in our society, increased imbalances are meted out from the **endocrine system** and, in particular, the thyroid. Because of its major influence on the whole body as well as its sensitivity in scale, the thyroid earned itself third place in the intermedial hierarchy. However, we cannot separate the parathyroid reflex from the thyroid reflex. Similar to the Pituitary / Pineal dominant reflexes – if you work one, you are working the other.

Parathyroid

The **parathyroid glands** are small endocrine glands in the neck that produce parathyroid hormone. We have four parathyroid glands, which are usually located on the posterior surface (back side) of the thyroid gland. The job of these glands is to maintain the body's calcium and phosphate levels within a very narrow range, so that the nervous and muscular systems can function properly. At the same time they do not allow the blood to carry off the calcium needed to support the density of bones. If someone has brittle bones or has kidney stones, look to the parathyroid reflex to unlock congestion that may be hindering its functions.

Performing the Thyroid / Parathyroid Reflexes

Anatomically the thyroid is inferior to the pituitary so we want to work at the base of the hallux to the most distal aspect to make sure that we strike not only the thyroid but the eyes, ears, head, sinus and parathyroids (see also the elementary reflexes on page 150 in Chapter Twelve 'Hierarchal Treatment: Elementary Reflexes to perform techniques for these associated reflexes using the index finger).

In *figure 11-3* I demonstrate how to use the thumb to drive the base flesh to reach the reflexes deeply. But the rest of the hallux can be worked with the index finger, as you'll note in the elementary reflexes.

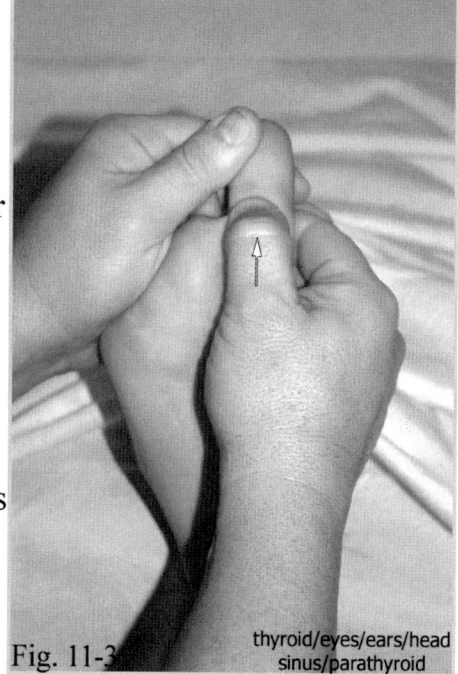

Fig. 11-3 thyroid/eyes/ears/head sinus/parathyroid

To do the thumb technique for the thyroid, start at the base of the first metatarsal head using your thumb to walk up the big toe – pausing halfway up and then starting again at the base, inching your way across, from medial to lateral as you move from proximal to distal. The holding hand's job is to hold the big toe firmly between the thumb and index finger so that pressure from the working hand's thumb does not cause the hallux to bend at the interphalangeal joint.

In other words, pressure from the holding hand's index finger must keep the hallux rigid and straight. It would be advisable to thumb-walk in many different directions in and around the base of the hallux to make sure that the thyroid area and associated members are struck with intensity.

Adrenals - the Fourth of the Intermedial Reflexes

The adrenal glands are two small endocrine glands – triangular in shape – that are located anterosuperiorly on the kidneys; perched on top of them, actually – one on each kidney. Two to three inches in length, each gland is comprised of a medulla (the center) and then surrounded by its cortex (or outer part of the gland). Both the **medulla** and **cortex** receive regulatory input from the nervous system (hypothalamus).

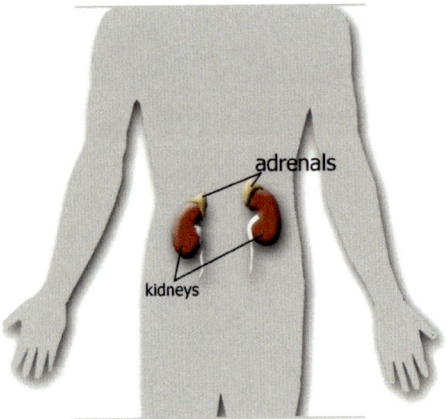

The **medulla** produces epinephrine (or adrenaline) and norepinephrine.

- **epinephrine** - also known as adrenalin. During the fight-or-flight response caused by the amygdala, the adrenal gland releases epinephrine into the blood stream (while the cortex pumps out other hormones like cortisol), signaling the heart to pump harder, increase blood pressure, open the airways in the lungs, narrow blood vessels in the skin and intestine to increase blood flow to major muscles, and performing other functions to enable the body to fight or run when encountering a threat. A healthy response in times of emergency, this system can go haywire, resulting in panic attacks; triggering these responses when there is no perceived threat. Adrenaline is an important activator on the Nervous System.
- **norepinephrine** – both a hormone and a neurotransmitter. It also directly increases the heart rate, stimulating the liver to release glucose from glycogen stores, and increasing blood flow to skeletal muscles. In its capacity as a hormone it teams up with epinephrine in the "fight or flight" response. As a neurotransmitter, it transmits nerve impulses from one neuron to the next.

The adrenal **cortex** produces other hormones necessary for fluid and **electrolyte** (salt) balance. It regulates water in the body and the blood that flows from the liver; along with helping control sugar metabolism and fighting inflammation in the body. It also supplements the sex hormones produced by the gonads. Let's look at just a couple of the hormonal functions:

- **cortisone** - is a steroid hormone. It is one of the byproducts of the process called steroidogenesis. This process starts with the synthesizing of **cholesterol,** followed by a series of processes in the adrenal gland to become any one of more than a few steroid hormones. Cortisone is also known as an anti-inflammatory.

Chapter 11 – Hierarchal Treatment: Intermedial Reflexes

- **cortisol** - small increases of this hormone have some positive effects: A quick burst of energy for survival reasons (working with epinephrine – as mentioned previously), heightened memory functions, a burst of increased immunity, lower sensitivity to pain, helps maintain homeostasis in the body.

Because of their incredible importance, they receive their rich blood supply from their own adrenal arteries. Because of their significance and their level of sensitivity, they've earned the fourth position of the intermedial hierarchal system.

Performing the Adrenal Reflexes

Holding the toes snug with the holding hand, use the working hand to drive the thumb in multiple directions between the Cuboid-Transverse guideline and the Cuboid-Oblique guideline as shown on *figure 11-4*. Even though the kidneys would lie medially, make sure to work the entire area in both feet.

You can cause greater sensitivity to the kidney reflex area by dorsal flexing the toes. Be careful of the flexor hallucis longus tendon when transversely working the area or while the toes are dorsally flexed. Try to skip over the tendon so as not to bruise it.

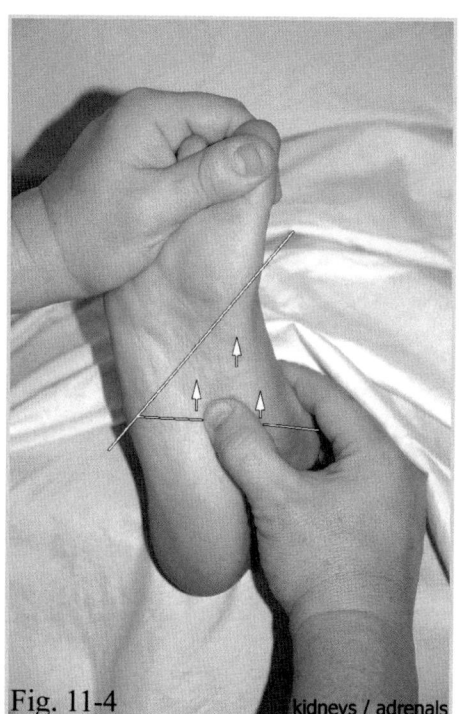

Fig. 11-4 kidneys / adrenals

Chapter 11 – Hierarchal Treatment: Intermedial Reflexes

Pancreas – the Fifth of the Intermedial Reflexes

The pancreas is a dual-function organ with both **endocrine** (glands of internal secretion in the bloodstream) and **exocrine glands** (glands of external secretion outside the bloodstream) that is sorely needed for the health and homeostasis of our makeup.

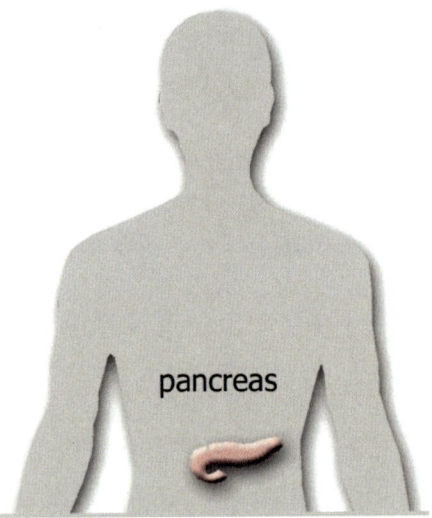

The pancreas is mostly composed of exocrine tissue for the digestive system, and secretions from those cells flow into a series of ducts for delivery into the **duodenum** (beginning of the small intestine). Sparsely scattered within the exocrine tissue are clusters of endocrine cells that secrete hormones into the blood.

The easiest way for me to describe the functions of the pancreas is to break the organ into two parts. Let's first look at the endocrine aspect. The major endocrine hormones that the pancreas secretes - insulin and glucagon - play a vital role in carbohydrate and lipid metabolism, necessary for maintaining normal blood sugar levels and staving off Type II Diabetes (adult onset).

Homeostasis requires blood sugar to be maintained in a very narrow range. Insulin and glucagon are the hormones that perform this function. It is the production of insulin and glucagon by the pancreas which ultimately determines if a patient has diabetes, hypoglycemia, or some other sugar problem. They are both secreted in response to blood sugar levels, but act as a counterbalance to one another.

Insulin: A proteinaceous hormone secreted by the **islets of langerhans** within the pancreas' exocrine tissue. Insulin is secreted into the bloodstream to activate cells in the absorption of **glucose** from digested carbohydrates (or sugars) in the blood. If an individual does not secrete enough insulin then blood sugar levels rise causing diabetes (high blood sugar). When too much insulin is released, sugar is rapidly removed from the blood to a detrimental degree, causing a hypoglycemic attack (low blood sugar).

Glucagon: Glucagon works in much the same manner as insulin...except in the opposite direction. If blood glucose is high, then no glucagon is secreted. When blood glucose goes LOW, however, (from lack of food or vigorous exercise), glucagon is secreted. The effect of glucagon is to make, most notably, the liver release the glucose (sugar) it has stored in its cells into the blood stream. This has the effect of increasing blood sugar.

As **chyme** (semi-digested food) floods into the small intestine from the stomach, two things have to happen: One is that the acid must be quickly and efficiently neutralized to prevent damage to the **mucosa** (myou-**koh**-suh) of the duodenum. In other words, acid from the stomach, if not neutralized by higher pH material, will allow for the scarring of the inner lining membrane of the small intestines. Bile from the gallbladder along with the pancreatic juices, which consist of digestive enzymes and bicarbonate, neutralize this acid at the beginning of the duodenum.

The other is that the macronutrients - proteins, fats and starches - must be broken down much further before their components can be absorbed through the mucosa of the **jejunum** (ji-**jew**-num) and ileum of the small intestine and then into the bloodstream.

These vital roles of the pancreas along with the sensitivity on the pain scale place this organ as the fifth of the intermedial reflexes.

Performing the Pancreatic Reflexes

The Cuboid Oblique guideline is designed to give you a general idea of where the pancreas / spleen reflex is located. This is not a perfect location rather a guide to the general understanding of the anatomical positioning as a reference. If you strike transversely and obliquely across the cuboid-oblique line from either direction (medial to lateral or vice versa) or posterior to anterior across the plantar surface, you should be able to reach these reflexes. In the left foot you would be striking the pancreas / spleen and in the right foot you would be hitting the liver / gallbladder. Use these instructions for either foot.

Firmly hold the toes with the holding hand as you drive your hand with the working hand across the cuboid-oblique guideline as seen in *figure 11-5*. Make several passes transecting the cuboid-oblique guideline in all directions. Drive the thumb as deeply as possible into the tissue while torquing the feet with the holding hand.

Chapter 11 – Hierarchal Treatment: Intermedial Reflexes

Liver – the Sixth of the Intermedial Reflexes

The largest solid organ of the body, only second to the skin, is the liver which weighs approximately 3.5 pounds and measures about 8 inches in length, 6.5 inches in height and about 4.5 inches thick.

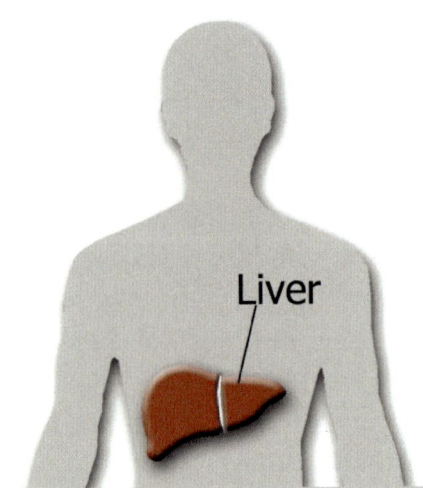

This incredible marvel has well over 500 functions and is known as 'the laboratory of the human body'. It has been postulated by many in the scientific community that the liver is connected to, or is at least aware of, every disease or dysfunction going on inside the body. I cannot even begin to scratch the surface in this book on the many functions of this organ. However, we can touch on just a few:

- Detoxifies the blood of all metabolic wastes (toxins like ammonia) and other exogenous (ex-aw-gen-us) substances, such as: drugs, alcohol and environmental toxins.
- Creates proteins to help maintain the volume of blood and factors in blood-clotting. The liver stores blood and regulates the volume of blood circulation according to the needs of various tissues and organs. When the body is at rest the amount of blood it requires decreases and the surplus is stored in the liver. During vigorous activity blood is released from the liver to increase the volume of circulating blood.
- Breaks down and stores carbohydrates for future use by the pancreas for energy levels in the body.
- Makes, stores and metabolizes fats, including fatty acids either as energy or acid neutralizers or cholesterol. By the way, I believe that most of our sicknesses today are acid-based and that high cholesterol is simply a symptom of too much acid in the blood.
- Forms and secretes bile to aid in the intestinal absorption of fats and the fat-soluble vitamins A, D, E, and K. Bile acts as one of the first hydrochloric acid neutralizers from the stomach, through the bile duct into the duodenum.
- Converts **lactic acid** from waste to storage fuel. Lactic acid is produced when glucose is metabolized through the energy production cycle (exercising your muscles). When excessive levels accumulate, muscle cramping can occur. A healthy liver will extract lactic acid from the bloodstream and convert it into the reserve endurance fuel, glycogen (stored glucose).

This marvelous organ along with its sensitivity on the pain scale puts it at the sixth spot on the Intermedial Hierarchy.

Performing the Liver Reflexes

Refer back to 'Performing the Pancreatic Reflexes' on page 140 of this chapter for instructions on how to perform the Liver Reflex techniques. See *figure 11-6* as it shows the location of the reflexes. Remember: it is simply the opposite of the pancreas on the oppositional foot.

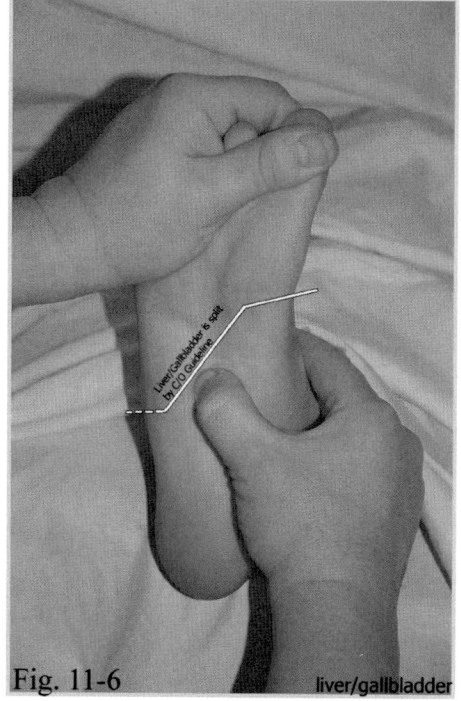

Fig. 11-6 liver/gallbladder

Kidneys – the Seventh of the Intermedial Reflexes

As reflexologists, we must be keenly aware of the need of the body to rid itself of toxins. After all, that is the staple of our modality through the striking of reflexes.

Most people look to the liver when they have toxic issues, but we should also look at our filter friends, the kidneys.

The kidneys are located in the posterior part of the abdominal cavity. There are two, one on each side of the spine; the left one lies posterior to the spleen, the right kidney lies posterior to the liver. Each kidney size is approximately 3.5" to 5" inches in diameter.

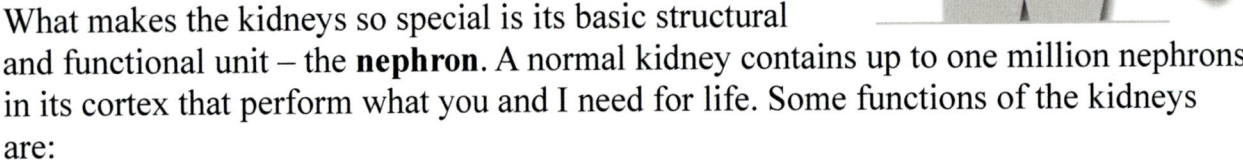

The kidneys are known as the 'Master Chemists' of the body but should also be known for their irreplaceable role as the 'Master Filters' of the body.

What makes the kidneys so special is its basic structural and functional unit – the **nephron**. A normal kidney contains up to one million nephrons in its cortex that perform what you and I need for life. Some functions of the kidneys are:

- regulates the concentration of water and soluble substances like sodium salts, by filtering the blood and eliminating waste as urine
- manages the pH of the blood (the acid or alkalinity of the blood)
- regulates blood pressure
- adjusts blood volume
- controls electrolytes
- removes uric acid
- removes excess calcium
- removes toxins

The endocrine system maintains strong control over the kidneys. One example is the parathyroids' control of calcium in the blood by stimulating the kidneys to either hold or eliminate calcium in the blood. Therefore, it is important to work the kidney reflex as well as the parathyroid to maintain calcium balance of the body.

If the nephrons do not receive enough water (because of inadequate water intake) then we may see conditions like **kidney stones** develop because of the clogging of the nephrons. Remember, the kidneys can amazingly filter up to 15 gallons of blood an hour which requires a lot of water for the removing of toxins.

Because of their importance in the sustaining of life, along with their intensity when worked, I give the **kidneys** the **seventh position** on the Intermedial Hierarchy.

Performing the Kidney Reflexes

Refer back to 'Performing the Adrenal Reflexes' on page 138 of this chapter for instructions on how to perform the Kidney Reflex technique.

****

In the final analysis, the intermedial reflexes open the way for the elementary reflexes to be stimulated and determine, once again, who is in charge of the health exercise.

Chapter Twelve

Hierarchal Treatment:

The Elementary Reflexes

Hierarchal Treatment – Elementary Reflexes

In this chapter we will discuss how to perform the Elementary reflex techniques and an explanation as to how these reflexes affect the hierarchy and value to the entire physiological association. I would like you to note that I do not give a specific order as to how these reflexes affect the other elementary reflexes. After years of study it became apparent that dominant and intermedial reflexes were easily exposed because of my **sensitivity scale**, which just happened to coincide with the value of that vital, with regards to how it related to relaxation and detoxification of oneself.

Even though these reflexes are important to all of our life's functions I could not determine what has greater importance over another. The sensitivity scale, as well as client feedback, deemed these reflexes as minor – as to the entire body's association of reflexes and the effect it had on each client. In other words, by the time all of the dominant and intermedial reflexes have been struck with sensitivity and have submitted to the reflexologist's request, the elementary reflexes join in line without resisting. **Only the most acute issue found in and among the elementary reflexes can seem to make this observation wrong.**

One false alarm is the misunderstanding of the reflex that corresponds to the heart and breasts. Reflex pain in this area has led the client and reflexologist to wonder if there is an issue with the heart, breasts or lungs. Here is a good reason why reflexologists should never diagnose. Why? Because the most likely condition is one of the metatarsals and its joints at the phalanges' base. Refer to Chapter Four – 'Conditions of the Feet' to get an idea as to how shoes and surfaces we walk on can cause terrible pain in the feet.

A reflexologist must be able to discern what the pain is from: from improper shoes, or reflex pain, and / or pain from real congestion in the feet (like uric acid) in order for the reflexologist to adjust pressure. Due to the fact that most new clients have a lot of congestion in their feet on the first visit, it takes several visits to make these findings. Information from their doctor, along with their own testimony of their health will either solidify your science or open new challenges to your art. This is a learning process with no end in sight. So be patient with yourself as well as your client's needs.

With this said, the elementary reflexes lack the intensity of their higher-tiered brothers, thus putting them in this category.

Chapter 12 – Hierarchal Treatment: Elementary Reflexes

The Sinus, Head, Eyes, Ears Reflexes

Sinus

Paranasal sinuses are air-filled spaces, communicating with the nasal cavity within the bones of the skull and face. The skull contains 4 major pairs of hollow air-filled sacks that connect the space between the nostrils and the nasal passage. Sinuses help insulate the skull, reduce its weight, and allow the voice to resonate within it.

Here are the four basic areas where the sinuses are located:

- Sphenoid sinuses (behind the eyes)
- Ethmoid sinuses (between the eyes)
- Frontal sinuses (in the forehead)
- Maxillary sinuses (behind the cheek bones)

These sinuses are covered with a mucus layer and cells that contain little hairs called cilia on their surface. These help trap and force bacteria and toxic pollutants outwardly. However, when the tissue becomes overwhelmed by bacteria - infection can set in. Acute sinusitis can also be caused by allergens (allergy-causing substances) or pollutants.

Some of my clients tell me that it feels like their head is going to explode. No matter how hard they blow their nose, more fluid fills the cavity. They are the lucky ones. Some clients have such acute inflammation they cannot get any air in through the nose.

It is a shame that the body's defenses become hypersensitive causing misery to the client. Try and bring them relief by striking as many reflexes as possible. They have some major blockages somewhere and we must do our best to get the brain to work on these issues.

Head

When working the head area we would also be working many other reflexes. But, we should cover every area of the head reflex to make sure that all tissue, muscle, and other physiology is normalized for homeostasis.

Eyes

If I had a scale for importance alone, the eyes would take the prize. Who would trade another body member for the eyes? The eyes play a vital role as a sense organ, giving us vision of our surroundings and putting images to the sounds we have come to know. The eyes can bring many sight blessings when they are working properly. Think about it, you're reading this using your eyes and hopefully not while you're driving your car.

The brain "sees" objects with a process started by the eyes. The things we see are a result of the light waves coming from an object. That is why we cannot sense objects visually when light is absent.

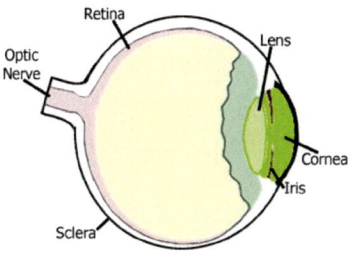

The Eye

Here are the stages of how light can be interpreted by the brain:

- Light enters first through the **cornea** (the clear dome in the front of the eye).
- Then it goes through the **pupil** (the opening in the center of the **iris** which is the colored part of the eye).
- The amount of light coming into the eye will cause the pupil to constrict, allowing or reducing incoming light.
- The cornea bends the light waves and they are then further bent by the **lens** (which is right behind the iris and pupil).
- The waves converge to a **nodal** point at the back surface of the lens, where the image is reversed (backwards) and inverted (or upside-down).
- The **vitreous humor**, a clear gel-like tissue that comprises most of the eye, allows the light to continue to the **retina**.
- The retina processes this light into electrical signals, sending them through the optic nerve to be interpreted by the brain – where we "see" the image.

Ears

You're probably familiar with the trite phrase, 'You don't know what you got until it's gone.' Even famous rock stars sing about it. For those that experience hearing loss, that statement rings so true (no pun intended). Not only do our ears bring us joy by letting us hear music, either from man or nature, but facilitate communication and alert us to danger. The ears are major parts of our auditory sense. They also help the body to maintain equilibrium (balance).

Chapter 12 – Hierarchal Treatment: Elementary Reflexes

The human ear consists of three parts:

- The outer ear (or visible portion), which includes the auricle (the skin covered flap) and the auditory canal (the opening which leads to the eardrum).
- The middle ear, which contains three small bones: the malleus (shaped like and referred to as a 'hammer'), the incus (like an anvil) and stapes (similar to stirrups). The middle ear is separated from the outer by the eardrum and air penetrates it by moving the auditory tube (Eustachian) which connects it to the throat.
- The inner ear (labyrinth) is comprised of the cochlea and the vestibule. The cochlea contains the sound-analyzing cells while the vestibule houses the organs that affect equilibrium.

In the process of hearing:

- Sound waves enter the auditory canal and hit the eardrum, causing vibrations. These waves pass from the larger surface area of the eardrum to the small opening of the inner ear.
- The vibration of the stapes (or stirrups) in the inner ear sets in motion the fluid of the cochlea.
- Changes in pressure stimulate a membrane which in turn moves the hair cells located in the cochlea.
- The sensory hair cells send impulses along the auditory nerve to the brain.

Maintaining balance seems to be a growing concern among the older population. Many begin losing their orientation, placing themselves in danger of injury to self and others. One of my clients cannot sleep lying down horizontally because that causes waves of dizziness to the point of vomiting. It's a feeling of being on a wayward ship on the high seas.

The ears are not only for hearing. They contain organs that help us to maintain our balance. The inner ear contains:

- The **utriculus** (you-**trick**-you-lus) and the **sacculus** (**sack**-you-lus)– the main organs determining orientation and balance.
- Three fluid-filled semicircular canals. Two of these canals determine vertical body movements and the third determines horizontal movements.

Whether we're jumping, running, sleeping or on a roller coaster, fluid moves back and forth over sensory hair cells in the canals or a gelatinous substance with lime crystals with regards to the utriculus and sacculus that tell the brain, through the auditory nerve, where we are in orientation. If all is working properly, our position should not have to be consciously considered but be autonomic.

However, some develop issues that make it difficult to stay balanced or feel balanced and oriented to the point where their life is affected. Some cannot: ride in the back of a car, go boating, ride certain rides at a theme park, swing or do the merry-go-round at a playground. In more extreme circumstances, some cannot: ride an elevator, walk up the stairs, swim or even lie down to sleep.

Performing the The Sinus, Head, Eyes, Ears Reflex

Split the holding hand over the toes with the thumb on the plantar aspect of the hallux and the index finger on the dorsal side as shown in *figure 12-1*.

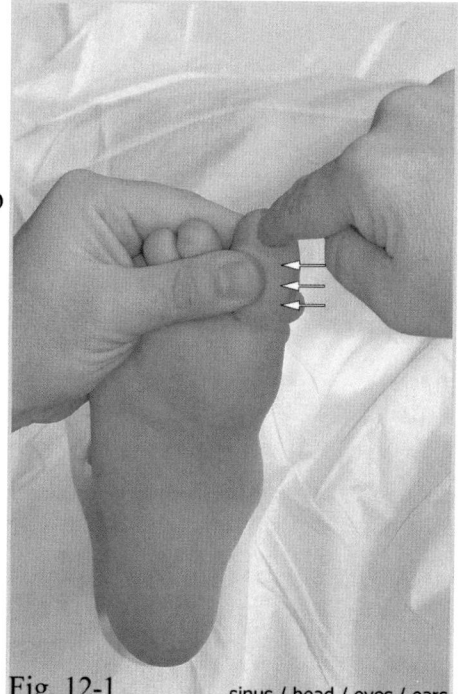

Use the index finger of the holding hand as leverage against the index finger of the working hand. The thumb of the holding hand should move as the index finger from the working hand moves medial to lateral across the entire plantar surface of the hallux.

The index finger of the working hand rolls in tiny 'bites' across the skin surface of the hallux. It is important that you keep the index finger of the working hand rigid and straight as you make these tiny, driving motions.

The motions should come from the wrist of the working hand. This technique is a perfect example of why you need to keep your nails cut short. We would not want to have our nail cut into their skin!

Fig. 12-1 sinus / head / eyes / ears

Chapter 12 – Hierarchal Treatment: Elementary Reflexes

The Heart, Pectoralis Major, Ribs, Esophagus, Bronchial, Breasts Reflexes

Heart

The heart has been referred to as the body's "engine room", responsible for pumping approximately five quarts of blood every minute throughout the body's circulatory system. Our network of blood vessels, which is comprised of arteries, veins and capillaries, is over 60,000 miles long and by the end of our lifetime would have probably clocked three billion heartbeats.

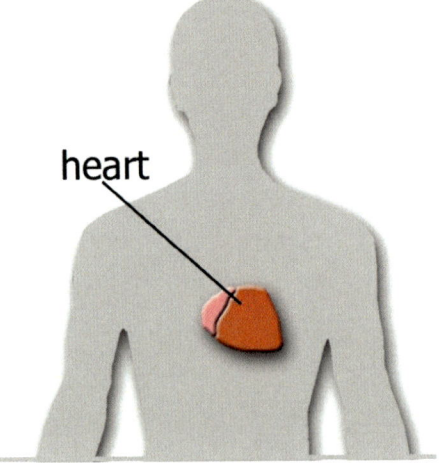

Located in the center of the chest between the lungs and sitting behind the breastbone and protectively ensconced in the confines of the ribcage, the heart supplies the body with oxygen and nutrients while also getting rid of wastes. The heart delivers oxygen from the lungs to the other organs and tissues and also removes carbon dioxide to the lungs where it's expelled.

Blood, pumped by the heart, not only oxygenates the organs and tissues, but delivers nourishment from the digestive system and hormones from the body's glands. Our immune system is also dependent on this since immune system cells travel in the blood, speeding waste products to the endocrine system to be dealt with.

The heart is a four-chambered organ about the size of a clenched fist. It's made up of cardiac muscle that works involuntarily. Under normal conditions, the heart beats (contracting and relaxing) from 70 to 80 times each minute. Each heart beat fills all four of the chambers with fresh blood. The four cavities form two separate pumps. These two pumps are divided by the septum (a wall of muscle). The **atria** (plural for atrium) are the upper chambers for each of these pumps, connected by a sealing valve to the **ventricles**, which are the larger, stronger portion of each of the pumps. Each time the heart contracts, the chambers force blood out of the atria and into the ventricles. The blood then travels from each ventricle into a large blood vessel at the top of the heart.

There are two main arteries at the top of the heart. The **pulmonary artery** speeds blood to the lungs to be oxygenated while the other, the **aorta**, delivers the oxygenated blood to the rest of the body. Veins are the vessels that bring blood to the heart. The two main veins are called the **vena cava**.

The heart is clearly a miraculous and essential organ and, unfortunately, heart disease is at this time the leading cause of death for both men and women in the United States. It is believed that the several types of heart disease, in many cases, are due to changes in lifestyle and diet. Hypertension and diabetes contribute to heart problems while others develop an arrhythmia, murmur, or irregular heartbeat. These heart problems can greatly affect one's lifestyle. While a heart attack is sudden, its causes are not. It is the course of wisdom to take care of the heart since, like most organs, it's the only one we have.

Pectoralis Major

The Pectoralis Major (also known as 'pecs') is a dense, fan-shaped muscle, located at the anterior (upper front) of the chest wall. It makes up the biggest share of the chest muscles and, in females, lies under the breasts. This major muscle is responsible for many lifting assignments and sports actions such as baseball. This is because of how it controls the actions of the **humerus** (large bone in the arm).

Ribs

The ribs form a protective cage around the vitals of the upper body, giving the chest its familiar shape.

They also hold up all the muscles of the upper torso. They're attached directly to the spine, but do not necessarily attach to the sternum in front or other ribs in the front.

These 24 bones, arranged 12 per side, are divided into three categories:

- The **True Ribs** are the first seven bones. They connect to the spine and the sternum by the costal cartilage.
- The **False Ribs** are connected to the spine but only attach to the lowest true rib in front and not the sternum.
- The **Floating Ribs** are the last two sets and are referred to as such because they are attached to the spine only, not connected to anything in front.

Esophagus

The esophagus is an organ which consists of a muscular tube through which food passes from the **pharynx (fair-inks)** to the stomach. Food is passed through the esophagus by the process of **peristalsis** (pair-i-**stall**-sis). The esophagus is lined with muscle that acts with peristaltic action (contracts much like a snake) to move swallowed food down to the stomach.

Bronchial

In each of the two lungs are the bronchus branches; which are airways inside the lungs. Each of the **bronchi**, which are connected to the trachea (or windpipe), divide many times – fractionally branching into smaller and smaller bronchi. These bronchi then branch into **bronchioles** – the smallest and narrowest airways.

The bronchi with its branches are referred to as the "bronchial tree" since they resemble an upside-down tree. The bronchi have cartilage, smooth muscle and mucus-secreting glands in its linings. The cartilage holds open the airways and the muscles cause the airways to dilate or constrict. The tiny bronchioles punctuating the bronchial branches have thousands of small air sacs called **alveoli** (al-**vee**-o-lie).

The bronchi are important parts of the lungs to strike when working reflexes as many people suffer from bronchial problems. **Bronchitis** is a condition where the air passages (the windpipe and the bronchi) become inflamed due to infection or pollutants. It manifests itself with symptoms including coughing, expectorating mucus – sometimes with blood, wheezing, nasal congestion / runny nose as well as swelling in the bronchial tubes and bronchioles and alveoli.

Bronchitis can become Acute Bronchitis if it's a secondary infection, preceded by a cold or influenza. If it is bacterial, antibiotics are often administered; but this difficult condition can be caused by the inhalation of fumes, dust, chemical solvents and tobacco smoke. If bronchitis is present for 3 months in two consecutive years, it's considered Chronic Bronchitis.

COPD or **Chronic Obstructive Pulmonary Disease** has Chronic Bronchitis as one of its subcategories. Since the main cause of COPD is smoking, this disease is preventative at least from that aspect. But bronchitis can be caused by colds or environmental allergens as well and should not be confused with **Bronchiolitis (bron**-kee-o-lie-tis)– the inflammation of the bronchioles caused by a virus more common in infancy.

Breasts

The breasts of a female are known for secreting milk for nourishing a child. They also contain lymph nodes that handle drainage. This is particularly relevant to oncology since breast cancer is a common cancer. When cancer metastasizes, wayward cancer cells break free from a tumor and spread to other parts of the body through the lymph system.

Performing the Heart, Pectoralis Major, Ribs, Esophagus, Bronchial, Breasts Reflexes

The holding hand should hold the toes snugly as the working hand's thumb drives the plantar surface from the cuboid oblique guideline to the clavicle guideline.

Use the forefingers of the holding hand to counter as leverage against the pressure of the working hand's thumb as seen in *figure 12-2*.

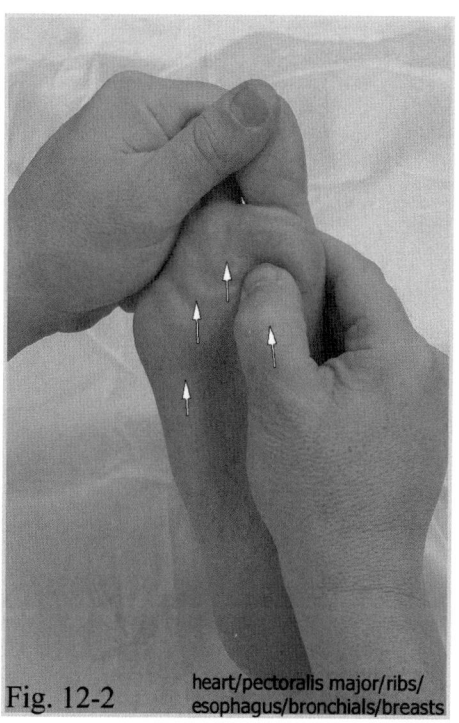

Fig. 12-2 heart/pectoralis major/ribs/esophagus/bronchials/breasts

As the thumb gets close to the fifth metatarsal head, the holding hand will need to be more active as the counter-lever. Make sure to drive deeply between the metatarsal bones to reach the deepest of reflexes.

The Deltoids Reflexes

The deltoid muscle is the muscle forming the rounded contour of the shoulder and has three parts: Anterior Fibers, Posterior Fibers and Lateral (middle) Fibers. The deltoid functions by rotating the arm in many directions assisting one to perform many daily functions. Most people complain of shoulder pain and shoulder injuries in and around the deltoid. Sometimes the deltoid can be the problem that issues the pain, however, generally it is the bicep attachment, triceps attachment or rotator cuff that is the issue and not the deltoid itself.

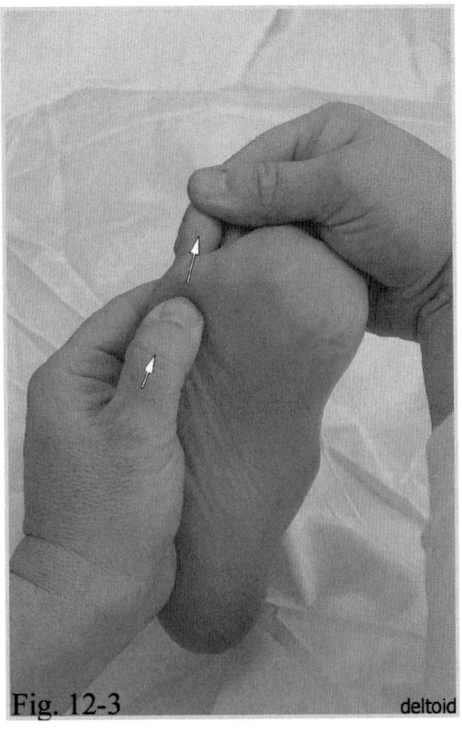

Fig. 12-3   deltoid

I use the deltoid as a line of demarcation on my chart that gives reference to all issues in and around the deltoid. Remember that the chart is designed to give a reference point only. It would be proper to describe to the client that you are working in and around the deltoid which includes the rotator cuffs, bicep and triceps attachments, and all ligament and tendon structures.

Performing the Deltoids Reflexes

The palm of the holding hand must securely hold the hallux as the thumb and the index finger grip the fifth digit so that the thumb of the working hand can drive up the phalanges of the fifth digit.

Use the holding hand to dorsal flex all the toes back to really get the thumb of the working hand in there between the fourth and fifth digits as evidenced in *figure 12-3*. Work anterior, posterior and lateral aspects of the deltoid region to ensure that all members are reached.

Focus on the lateral aspect by using the index finger of the working hand to strike the most lateral part of the phalanges of the fifth digit. Work from the head of the fifth metatarsal all the way to the tip of the fifth digit's toe using the index finger to reach this crucial reflex.

The Stomach Reflex

The stomach is part of the digestive system and is attached on the superior end to the esophagus and on the inferior end to the **duodenum** (doo-uh-**dee**-num). The stomach cannot be accurately sized from a homogeneous (huh-**maw**-jen-us) standpoint because its size depends upon how much one eats, although estimates are six to eight inches.

When it's empty, an adult's stomach has a volume of one-fifth of a cup, but it can expand to hold more than eight cups of food after a large meal. The stomach is affected by how well the food is masticated (chewed) and saturated with saliva.

The stomach can be divided into two regions: a reservoir and a grinder. The upper stomach (the reservoir) stores the masticated food. The lower stomach (the grinder) develops strong peristaltic waves of contraction that mixes the food with gastric juices.

The gastric juices include hydrochloric acid, pepsin and other powerful enzymes needed to break down the complex proteins and other elements into a soluble fluid. These powerful contractions constitute a very effective gastric grinder, occurring about 3 times per minute.

The gastric juices are produced by tiny glands in the walls lining the stomach. Hydrochloric acid is so powerful it could burn a hole in your couch, so why doesn't it dissolve your stomach? Your stomach also produces a mucus that protects the walls from this acid. It is truly remarkable.

Some substances, such as water, salt, sugars, and alcohol can be absorbed directly through the stomach wall. That's why diabetics or those that are dehydrated can restore their constitution quickly without the need for the general passing of nutrients that are absorbed through the entire alimentary (al-uh-**men**-tuh-ree) tract.

Most other substances in the food we eat need further digestion and must travel into the intestine before being absorbed.

Performing the Stomach Reflex

The stomach reflex is found in both feet between the cuboid-oblique guideline and the cuboid-transverse guideline. However, in the true anatomical position the stomach does cross the cuboid-oblique guideline laterally in the left foot. The image 'stomach' *figure 12-4* on page 157 shows the most extreme end of the reflex where it touches the guideline.

The holding hand should hold all toes snug as the working hand's thumb drives the flesh between the guidelines (see *figure 12-4*).

Make sure to work the most medial aspect which would cross the spinal reflex all the way up to the oblique guideline. I recommend that you work in all directions, switching hands.

On the right foot simply work between the guidelines.

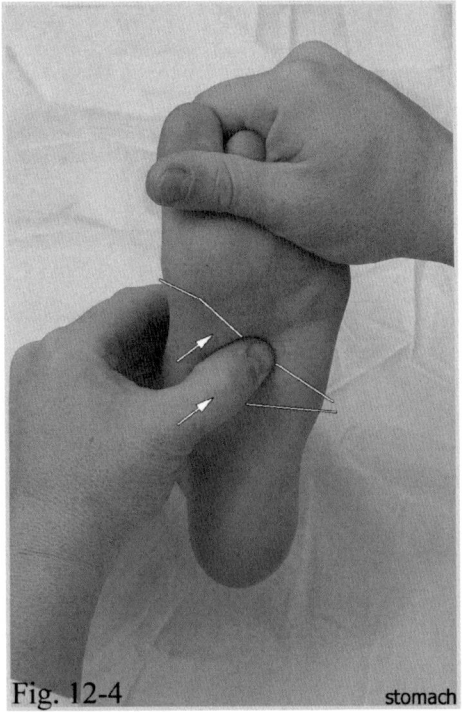

Fig. 12-4   stomach

The Gallbladder Reflexes

The gallbladder, in my opinion, is vital to good digestion, regardless of the fact that many seem to think you can just cut it out and be rid of it at the first sign of acute pain. Their reasoning is that the liver will do its job regardless. However, this four-inch organ is necessary in the storing of bile from the liver. It can store up to 1.7 ounces of bile that is secreted through a duct systematically to aid in neutralizing acids and digestion in the duodenum.

Bile concentrated in the gallbladder is more potent than the bile in the liver. This intensifies its effect on the emulsification of fats. Two thumbs up for the gallbladder!

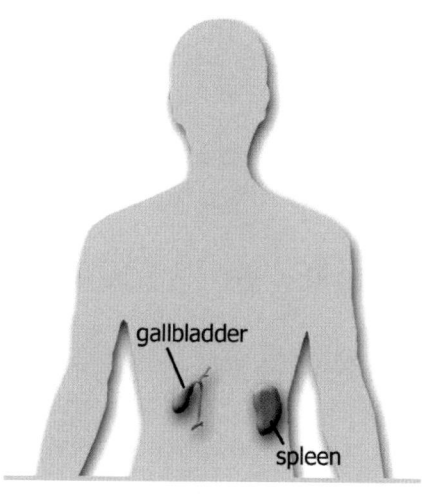

Performing the Gallbladder Reflexes

Look to the Liver Reflex Technique in Chapter Eleven 'Hierarchal Treatment: Intermedial Reflexes' on page 142.

The Spleen Reflex

The spleen, part of the lymphatic system, is in the uppermost area of the left side of the abdomen, just under the diaphragm. It has attachments to the stomach, left kidney, and colon and rests laterally to the pancreas. A primary function of the spleen is the production of antibodies while another responsibility is the filtration of worn-out red blood cells. Its role in immunity against bacterial infections involves the trapping of organisms with the white blood cells. The spleen is also a blood reservoir that supplies the body with blood in emergencies such as a bad cut.

Performing the Spleen Reflex

Because of the spleen's referral area, look to the Pancreas Reflex Technique in Chapter Eleven 'Hierarchal Treatment: Intermedial Reflexes' on page 140 to perform this reflex.

Chapter 12 – Hierarchal Treatment: Elementary Reflexes

The Arms, Hands, Elbows, Wrist, Biceps, Triceps Reflexes

Arms - The main bone of the arm is the humerus followed by the radius and the ulna in the lower arm.

Hands - As we know, the spine and feet have 26 bones each. But the hands have one extra carpal, containing 27 bones.

Biceps - A muscle located on the upper anterior aspect of the arm. The most important of its many functions are rotating the forearm and flexing the elbow. We use the bicep for just about everything.

Triceps - A set of three muscles on the posterior aspect of the arm that is used for extension of the elbow allowing one to push away from objects.

Performing the Arms, Hands, Elbows, Wrist, Biceps, Triceps Reflexes

This technique requires a lot of practice to improve upon the skill of 'walking' up the arm reflex with the working hand's thumb. Because of the soft tissue and the bony protrusion of the tuberosity of the fifth metatarsal bone, the thumb tends to deflect from its purposeful positioning and driving.

The holding hand must securely and firmly hold the foot from rotating while the pressure from the working hand is being used. In *figure 12-5*, you will notice the thumb driving deeply into the lateral flesh as the holding hand steadies the foot.

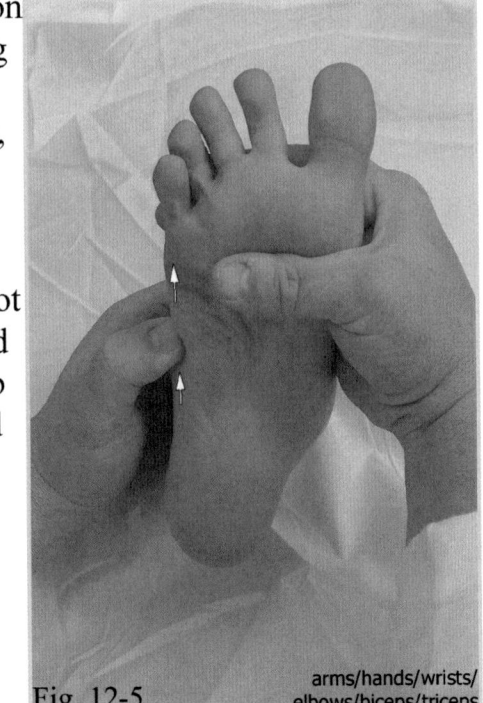

Fig. 12-5 arms/hands/wrists/elbows/biceps/triceps

Let the forefingers of the working hand slide up the dorsal aspect of the foot while rigid, yet not pinching. Your counter-leverage should come from the holding hand. Make sure to work the plantar, lateral and dorsal sides of the reflex to completely cover the arm and associated reflexes.

The Small Intestine, Colon, Bladder, Ureters, Testes, Ovaries, Uterus, Prostate Reflexes

Small Intestine

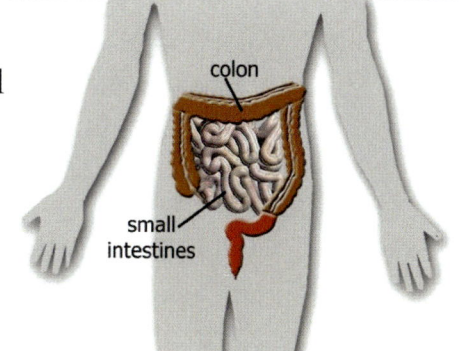

The small intestine is 23' feet in length and is called 'small' by virtue of the fact that the diameter of the small intestine is smaller than that of the large intestine. The small intestine is where nutrients are absorbed. The three sections of the small intestine are:

- The **Duodenum** (the beginning of the small intestine) is the shortest part and precedes the jejunum and the ileum. It is where most chemical digestion takes place and where it is critical that bile from the gallbladder mixed with digestive enzymes from the pancreas neutralizes the acid from the stomach.
- The **Jejunum** lies between the duodenum and the ileum and is referred to as the middle intestine. It absorbs nutrients from the gut contents.
- The **Ileum** is the final section of the small intestine. It mainly absorbs vitamin B12 and bile salts, and other nutrients not picked up by the jejunum.

After all absorption of nutrients, vitamins and minerals has taken place, the liquid that's left over passes through a sphincter valve (Ileocecal valve) at the end of the ileum that goes into the beginning of the ascending colon.

Colon

The colon is referred to as the large intestine because, although shorter than the small intestine at approximately five feet long, it is larger in diameter. The colon is known in six parts:

- The ascending colon (known as the cecum) extends from the Ileocecal valve to the hepatic flexure.
- The hepatic flexure (sharp turn by the liver)
- The transverse colon begins at the hepatic flexure and ends at the splenic flexure.
- The splenic flexure (sharp turn by the spleen)
- The descending colon begins at the splenic flexure and descends to the sigmoid colon.

- The sigmoid flexure is the sharp S-bend at the bottom and connects to the anus.

The large intestine is the terminus in the digestive tube and it functions in three processes:

1. It recovers water and electrolytes from **ingesta** (digestive tract material). About 90% of water is absorbed in the colon, with 10% being absorbed by the stomach walls.
2. As the water is removed, the liquid becomes more solid thus the creation of solid fecal matter. The dehydrated matter is mixed with bacteria and mucus to form the solid wastes before final elimination.
3. The large intestine is brimming with microbial life which produces enzymes for digesting what would otherwise be indigestible. *As a side note, many people who experience problems with digestion have found it beneficial to take probiotics in order to help the large intestines with this process.*

Bladder / Ureters

The bladder is the organ that collects urine excreted by the kidneys prior to disposal by urination. Urine enters the bladder via the ureters (ducts from the kidneys) and exits via the urethra (the tube that connects the bladder to the outside of the body).

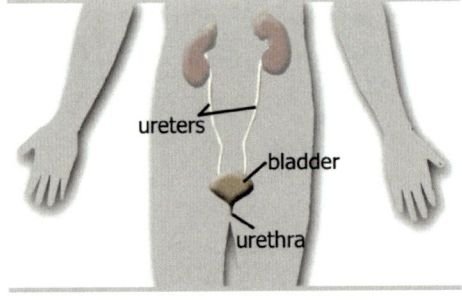

Testes

The testes (or testicles) are part of the male reproductive system. They consist of two oval organs about the size of large olives. Located inside the scrotum, the loose sac of skin that hangs behind the penis, the testes make the male hormones, including testosterone, and produce sperm, the male reproductive cells. Some disorders of the testes include hormonal imbalances, sexual dysfunction and infertility.

Prostate

The prostate is an exocrine gland of the male reproductive system. The main function of the prostate is to store and secrete a slightly alkaline fluid (thick and milky in appearance) that usually constitutes one-fourth of the volume of the semen along with sperm and seminal fluid. The prostatic fluid is expelled in the first ejaculate fractions together with most of the sperm. In comparison with the few sperm released with mainly seminal fluid – those expelled in prostatic fluid have better activity, longer survival and better protection of the DNA. The prostate also contains muscles that help expel semen during ejaculation.

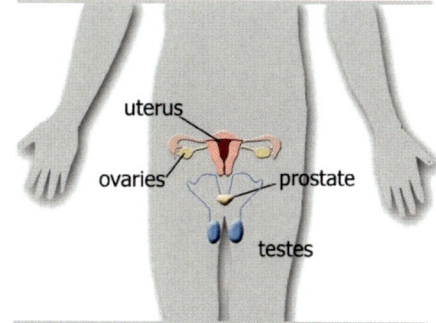

Ovaries

The ovaries are oval shaped, egg-producing reproductive organs about the size of olives. In pairs, corresponding to the testes in males, they are both gonadal and endocrine glands. Settled in front of the ureters, they are attached to the fallopian tubes. The ovaries generally take turns releasing the monthly eggs awaiting fertilization. The ovaries produce **estrogen** (**es**-tro-jen) and **progesterone** (pro-**jes**-tur-rone) in alternating phases of a woman's menstrual cycle.

Uterus

The uterus (womb) is a major female hormone-responsive reproductive sex organ. It is within the uterus that the fetus develops during gestation. One end of the uterus is the cervix which opens to the vagina. The other end is connected on two sides to the fallopian tubes, which in turn, connect to the ovaries.

The job of the uterus is to provide support to the bladder, bowel, pelvic bones and other organs. It is attached to bundles of nerves, arteries, veins and ligaments needed for various reasons including life support to a fetus. It also helps with uterine orgasm and is essential in sexual response since it directs blood flow to the pelvis and genitalia.

In its reproductive function, a fertilized ovum attaches itself to the uterine wall (the endometrium) and would be nourished by blood vessels specifically for this purpose. The zygote (fertilized egg) develops into a fetus and would continue to grow until childbirth. The uterus accepts a fertilized ovum which becomes implanted into the endometrium, and derives nourishment from blood vessels which develop exclusively for this purpose. The fertilized ovum becomes an embryo, develops into a fetus and gestates until childbirth.

Chapter 12 – Hierarchal Treatment: Elementary Reflexes

Performing the Small Intestines, Colon, Bladder, Ureters, Testes, Ovaries, Uterus, Prostate Reflexes

While holding the toes firmly with the holding hand (*see figure 12-6*), use the working hand to rotate the foot adduction as you drive the thumb from the working hand between the hip-sciatic guideline and the cuboid-transverse guideline.

The holding hand's palm should be over the lateral aspect of the foot at approximately the fifth metatarsal head. All the forefingers of the working hand slide around the ankle access from the medial to lateral aspect of the talus bone.

When working the bladder / ureters reflex make sure to drive your thumb along the medial plantar edge of the spinal reflex in that area. This would require you to cup the fingers underneath the ankle bone while driving the fingers vertically.

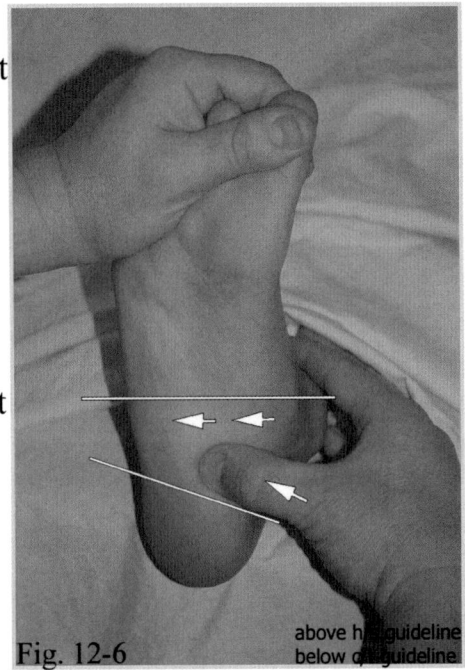

Fig. 12-6

above hip guideline
below cuboid guideline

Chapter 12 – Hierarchal Treatment: Elementary Reflexes

The Ileocecal Valve, Appendix Reflexes

The Ileocecal valve is a sphincter valve that separates the ileum (last part of the small intestine) from the cecum (beginning of the ascending colon). This sphincter muscle prevents fecal matter from the ascending colon to enter the ileum of the small intestine.

The problem is that refined food and stress can hinder this valve from closing all the way. Why does this matter? Because these toxic substances that seep back into the small intestine can cause bacterial infections that cause the body to produce a chemical called sterol to remove inflammation. These organic alcohols cause the body to overreact and produce chemicals such as tryptophan, which is a type of amino acid.

The body's reaction to this amino acid is to produce histamine, which is another amino acid that neutralizes tryptophan. And we all know what it means when there's a buildup of histamines in the body: sinus, bronchial and other allergic reactions.

The appendix lies about two centimeters below the Ileocecal valve and little is known about it. Some argue it serves no useful purpose while new studies believe it may have immunity functions.

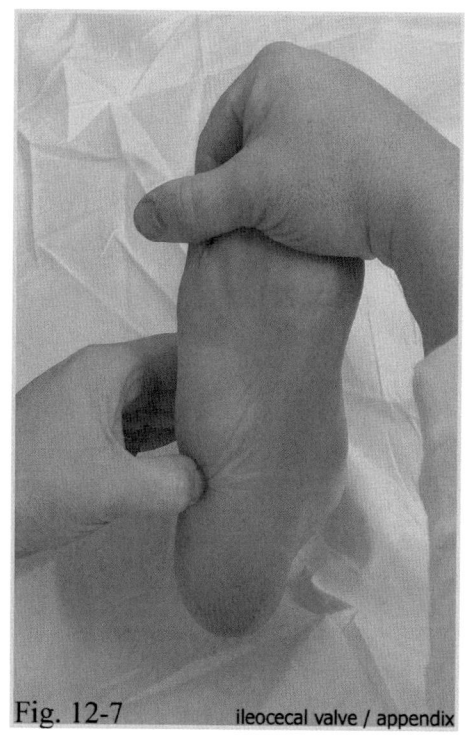

Fig. 12-7   ileocecal valve / appendix

Performing the Ileocecal Valve, Appendix Reflexes

Look at *figure 12-7* very closely and notice where the working hand's thumb is located. It's between the tuberosity of the fifth metatarsal base and the cuboid bone. We refer to it at a 'cuboid notch' or 'cuboid cushion' because it is the soft spot that the thumb seems to fit in perfectly.

Simply hook the thumb of the working hand in tiny 'bites' in and around this area. The holding hand should dorsal flex all the toes for maximum stretch.

Chapter 12 – Hierarchal Treatment: Elementary Reflexes

The Legs, Knees, Achilles Tendons, Gastrocnemius, Hamstrings, Quadriceps Reflexes

Legs

There are four bones in the leg: The femur, the tibia, the fibula and the patella.

The **femur** (**fee**-mur) is the largest bone in the body (and is the largest ball-and-socket joint as well). This upper leg bone connects the pelvis with the lower leg and forms the hip joint by articulating with the pelvis.

The **tibia** (**tib**-ee-yuh) is one of the two bones that make up the lower part of the leg and supports most of the body's weight.

The **fibula** (**fib**-yoo-luh) is the other of the two bones that make up the lower part of the leg and it provides support for the ankle as well as space for muscle attachments.

The **patella** (puh-**tell**-uh) is a small, triangular-shaped bone and is commonly referred to as the 'kneecap'.

The bones of the leg have very important functions. They allow rigidity for support and space for muscles, providing for a host of movements like running, kicking, jumping and lifting.

Knees

The knee joint is made up of three bones, a complicated series of ligaments and cartilage.

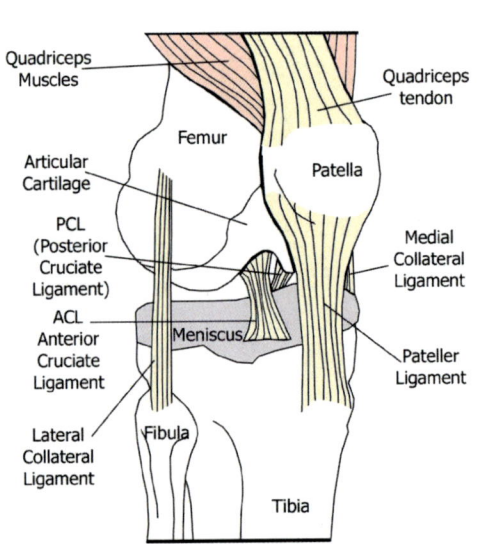

The knee is formed by the femur, the tibia, and the patella. Several muscles and ligaments control the motion of the knee, primarily the hamstrings and quadriceps, and allow us to do the activities we do. Because the knee is so complex, I thought I would share with you just some of the basic functions, so when your clients complain of knee pain, you might understand what they are talking about.

There are two major ligaments on either side of the knee, called the Medial and Lateral Collateral Ligaments, that stabilize the knee from side-to-side motions (medial to lateral). They help to keep the leg straight and allow for a swinging motion of the leg forward and backward.

There are two major ligaments inside the knee that stabilize it from pulling apart (from front-to-back) during normal activities. In other words, they keep the knee centered. The Anterior Cruciate (**crew**-shee-it) Ligament (commonly known as the 'ACL') is one of a pair of ligaments in the center of the knee joint that form a cross, and this is where the name "cruciate" comes from. There is also a Posterior Cruciate Ligament (commonly referred to as the 'PCL') which crosses the ACL.

These ligaments minimize the amount of wear and tear on the articular cartilage inside the knee which are directly attached to the bone. However, this cartilage would be very vulnerable if your body weight comes crashing down on it, bone-on-bone. So, thankfully, we have another type of cartilage that acts as a shock absorber called the meniscus (muh-**nis**-kiss). These two structures of cartilage are called the Medial Meniscus and the Lateral Meniscus.

The menisci (plural for meniscus / muh-**nis**-sky) are horseshoe-shaped shock absorbers that help to center the knee joint and minimize stress on the articular cartilage. The blending of the articular cartilage and the menisci creates an almost frictionless gliding surface.

Achilles Tendon

The Achilles is a large tendon that connects the gastrocnemius (calf muscle / gas-trok-**nee**-mee-us) to the calcaneus (heel bone / cal-**kay**-nee-us). It lets you rise up on your toes and push off when you walk or run. The explosive thrust of a sprinter is held together by this very important tendon.

In my experience, the working of the Achilles can be very tender. If the hamstrings and the calf muscle are tight, it will make the Achilles taut, like a group of guitar strings. It is more likely that the Achilles will tear under duress if the above condition exists. Make sure to work the area where the tendon meets the bone. It will stimulate relaxation of the tendon and the attached muscle.

Gastrocnemius

The gastrocnemius (**gas**-trok-**nee**-mee-us) is also known as the calf muscle. This muscle is used for stabilization in standing, running and jumping.

Hamstrings

The big group of muscles and tendons in the back of the thigh are commonly called the hamstrings. The role of the hamstring muscles is to bend (flex) the knee and to move the thigh backwards at the hip.

Quadriceps

The quadriceps are a group of four muscles that sit on the anterior or front aspect of the thigh. The function of the quadriceps as a whole is to extend the knee.

Performing the Legs, Knees, Achilles Tendons, Gastrocnemius, Hamstrings, Quadriceps Reflexes

Use the holding hand to secure the toes while dorsal flexing the foot with palm pressure on the metatarsal heads. Use the thumb of the working hand to drive into the plantar pad flesh as deeply as possible to affect this reflex (*see figure 12-8*).

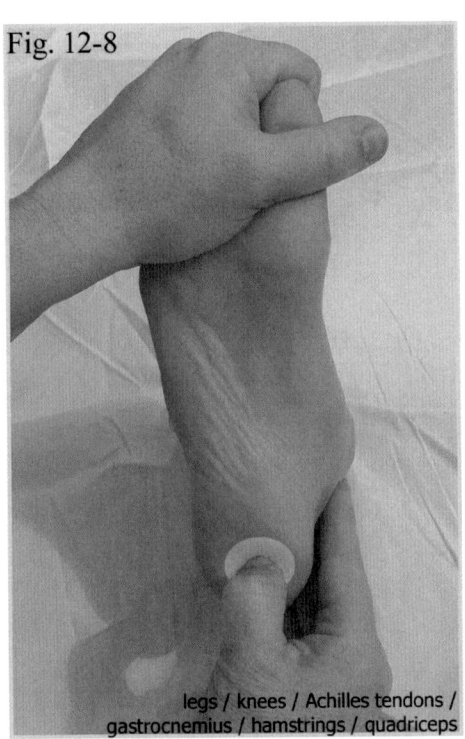

Fig. 12-8

legs / knees / Achilles tendons / gastrocnemius / hamstrings / quadriceps

The Clavicles Reflex

The clavicle (or collar bone) is a flat bone that makes up part of the pectoral girdle. The clavicle does the following:

- It serves as a rampart from which the scapula and free limb are suspended. This structure keeps the upper limb away from the thorax (upper torso) so that the arm has maximum range of motion.
- Transmits physical impacts from the upper limb to the axial skeleton (skull, ribs, spine and sternum).

Although classified as a 'long bone', the clavicle has no bone marrow cavity like other long bones. It is made up of spongy bone with a shell of compact bone. I use the clavicle bones as a guideline to separate the trapezius muscles from the pectoralis major on my chart and it makes for an excellent transverse guideline.

Performing the Clavicles Reflex

Simply strike in both directions the metatarsal heads across the clavicle guideline. This is a transverse striking of the reflex as well as vertically going between each of the metatarsal bones up to the phalanges. It's more of a guideline than an actual reflex, but we'll leave it at that.

The Sternum Reflex

The sternum is a flat bone located in the middle of the chest. The sternum, along with the ribs, forms the rib cage that protect the heart, lungs, and major blood vessels. The sternum is comprised of three parts:

- The **manubrium** (also called the "handle" / muh-**new**-bree-um) is located at the top of the sternum and articulates slightly. It has a connection to the first two ribs.
- The **body** (also called the "gladiolus") is located in the middle of the sternum and connects the third to seventh ribs directly. Indirectly it connects the eighth through tenth ribs.
- The **xiphoid process** (also called the "tip" / **zif**-oid) is located on the bottom of the sternum. It is often cartilaginous, but does become bony in later years. I like to use the xiphoid process as a marker to show where the beginning of the 'abdominal brain' begins.

These three sections of the bone are fused in adults. Costal cartilage connects the sternum to the ribs. The sternum protects the vitals and completes the ellipsis of the rib cage.

Performing the Sternum Reflex

When working the upper thoracics according to the spinal reflex techniques (see page 125 in Chapter Ten Hierarchal Treatment: Dominant Reflexes) you will be crossing over the sternum reflex. It's a good touchstone for location on the chart.

The Latissimus Dorsi Reflex

The latissimus dorsi is the larger, flat, postero-lateral muscle on the back, posterior to the arm, and partly covered by the trapezius on its median dorsal region (center region). It functions to help lift. When you deadlift (picking up something heavy right off the ground) you're using your 'lats'. When you row a boat, pull weeds, saw wood and do pull-ups, again, you're using your 'lats'. Without the lats, you would not be able to lift anything.

Performing the Latissimus Dorsi Reflex

This reflex is found on the dorsal side of the foot. It requires using the forefingers of the working hand to drive across the top of the foot from medial to lateral.

It's important to note that the fingers will want to glide over the metatarsal bones and not want to go in between the valleys. We must go in between each of the valleys by driving the fingers in to them between each of the bones.

You can do this transversely as in *figure 12-9* at right, or you can do this antero-posteriorly (vertically) from the toes down. Adjust the thumb pressure of the working hand so that the forefingers can dig properly into the dermis.

WARNING: Do not pull the foot towards you (plantar flexing the foot). In many cases it will cause discomfort because of its unnatural feeling and seems to cause cramping of the foot.

Fig. 12-9   latissimus dorsi

The Gluteus Maximus / Low Back Reflexes

The gluteus maximus is the largest of the three gluteal muscles. It makes up a large portion of the shape and appearance of the buttocks (nates / **nay**-teez). Its power is in the maintaining of the trunk in the erect posture.

Performing the Gluteus Maximus / Low Back Reflexes

To perform this reflex you must find the soft transition between the talus bone and the cuneiforms. Using a finger first probe around the transition of the dorsal flesh that folds when dorsal flexing the foot.

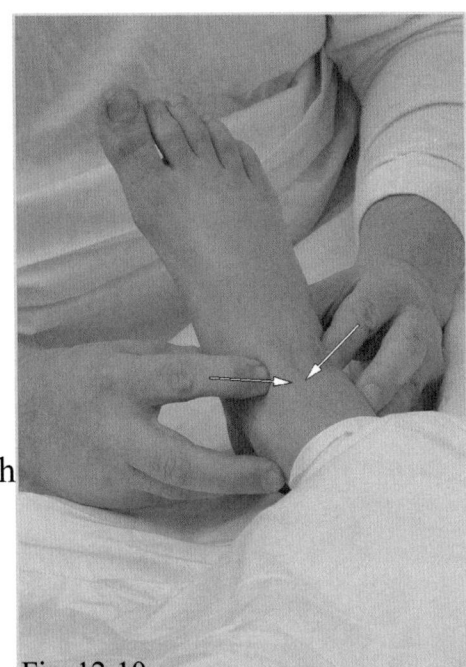

Fig. 12-10 gluteus maximus / low back

Once found, you can either use one index finger of a working hand to go medial-to-lateral, digging deeply through the valley; then switch hands and do the same. Or you can do as shown in *figure 12-10*. Use the index fingers of both hands at the same time to drive the dermis to hit the deepest part of the reflex.

****

After the reflexologist has done his best to strike the dominant, intermedial and elementary reflexes, it's up to the client's own body to do the rest and respond.

Chapter 12 – Hierarchal Treatment: Elementary Reflexes

Chapter Thirteen

The Lymphatic System

The Lymphatic System

The Lymphatic System is also referred to as the 'Immune System' of the body. It is called such because it functions to rid our body of toxic bacteria, fluids and worn-out cells that would lead to disease if not removed properly. Fluid leaks from tiny capillaries throughout the body. A system is needed to collect this fluid from the surrounding tissues so that it may be reused or removed from the body.

The Lymphatic System includes:
- Lymphatic organs such as the tonsils, thymus, and spleen.
- Isolated nodules of lymphatic groups in the intestinal wall.
- Lymph nodes located along the paths of collecting vessels.

The task of the lymphatic system is to transport the extra lymph fluid from the tissues and return it to the blood since, as mentioned earlier, the capillaries are constantly leaking fluids. This is necessary to keep the body from swelling with massive edema.

The immunity capabilities also work to protect the body from germs, viruses, fungi and bacteria that could make us ill. The lymph nodes, small masses of tissue located along the lymph vessels, filter out these germs. Lymphocytes are a type of white blood cell housed in the lymph nodes and some of these make antibodies to fight germs and check infection.

Tonsils and adenoids are the body's first line of defense. They sift through bacteria and viruses that enter the body through the mouth or nose at the risk of their own infection. The tonsils are soft tissue located on either side of the back of the mouth. Antibodies and immune cells in the tonsils help kill germs and help prevent throat and lung infections.

Adenoids are also made of glandular tissue, hanging from the upper part of the back of the nasal cavity. Like tonsils, adenoids help to defend the body from infection by trapping bacteria and viruses breathed in through the nose. They host cells and antibodies to help prevent throat and lung infections. Adenoids get bigger after birth but generally stop growing between the ages of 3 and 7 years.

The thymus is located just above the heart and grows rapidly from birth to puberty. Once sex hormones begin to be produced, it starts to shrink in size. It's task is to produce T-lymphocytes which help cells decipher enemy invaders in need of destruction for the body's survival.

The spleen also helps the body fight infection. The spleen contains lymphocytes and macrophages (**mac**-row-**faje**-is), another kind of white blood cell, which engulfs and destroys bacteria, dead tissue, and foreign matter and removes them from the blood passing through the spleen.

As reflexologists, we cannot pinpoint the entire lymphatic system through reflexes on a chart. However, as we work all the reflexes on the entire foot, we will reach all the elements of the lymphatic system. The only reflex of the lymphatic system that receives attention on the chart is the spleen. I left off the tonsils, adenoids and thymus because of the multiple overlapping reflexes in the corresponding referral areas. In other words, there is no sense in being specific about EVERY organ and gland or body part on the chart.

Chapter 13 – The Lymphatic System

Chapter Fourteen

Observations

Observations

Even though I do not keep records of observations anymore, I thought for the benefit of the readers, I would include some of my older observations based on dogmatic reflexes. My mind has changed on the dogma of fixed reflexes. My thinking has evolved on this matter as I've explained earlier in this book, as I've come to believe that there is a hierarchy to sensitive reflexes and extreme sensitivity is not always indicative of a problem in a particular area; although that MAY be the case – that extreme sensitivity will occur when there is an issue in a particular area. Depending on the point of view of the observations, some have been left in their original form, grammar issues and all.

Note:
*(SS) stands for Sensitivity Scale
*Scale goes from 1 to 10. 1 is like a light tickle and 10 feels like a nail is being driven into the foot. Reflex pain above a 7 gets my attention.

A Physician's Experience With Reflexology (First Person POV *[Point Of View]*)

"I'm a 56-year-old male physician. I experienced a severe, right knee sprain twenty years ago resulting in chronic knee pain. There are presently fascial contractions in my lower leg and hip that have developed. I've experienced mild lower back pain and right mid-foot and heel pain for two years as well as stiffness in the right knee/foot and noticeable stiffness in my gait; frequent stretching is no longer working. Also, neck pain associated with sinus drainage."

1st treatment: Sharp pains in both feet, the right one most severe during treatment. I experienced heat "flush" in right neck and enjoyed five days of nasal passage relief following treatment. After treatment, both feet felt like I was walking on air cushions, which continued for two to three days. Right foot pain was gone for five days. Only mild, mid-foot pain returned. A feeling of incredibly deep relaxation for thirty minutes after treatment and a tranquil state that lasted for several hours.

2nd and 3rd treatments: Much less tenderness in feet during treatment. Intense heat flushes to face and chest during mid-treatment, especially to right side of neck. Walking on air cushion sensation following treatment six days. Foot pain did not return. Noticed flexibility had returned to knee and walked without stiffness in gait. Neck issue was 99% gone since the third treatment. Deep relaxation after treatment and tranquil state lasted for about one hour.

Chapter 14 - Observations

4th treatment: No tenderness in feet during treatment. Walking on air feeling lasted six days. I experienced mild, mid-foot discomfort on seventh day. Right knee ache gone (had been chronic for twenty years). No tenderness in knee to deep rubbing. Neck pain still gone. My right foot was feeling very flexible. I had less 'heat' sensations in this treatment. I experienced less profound relaxation, but still long-lasting tranquility (less irritability). In the last ten minutes of treatment, I felt my right lung fill with mucus, which expelled frequently in the next sixty minutes; also a great deal of intestinal 'growling' during the last half of treatment. Experiencing no NP or foot pain at all. Air cushion effect continues.

5th treatment: Entered treatment with no pain in body, but tired after a hard day. No foot pain during treatment except very tender in adrenal region of right foot. During treatment heartbeat strength and noted increase which continued six hours after treatment. Also experienced an agitated, nervous state which lasted for several hours; unable to 'wind down'. Slept well and awoke refreshed and normal. Air cushion in feet remains.

6th treatment: No body pain entering treatment. My feet were not tender nor was there any heat sensation during treatment. I experienced an odd right, mid-foot sensation near little toe-side during treatment and I also felt deep relaxation following it and a tranquil attitude for a short time. The air cushion sensation and youthful "spring in my step" feeling lasted for several hours following reflexology.

Results so far:
1) No more Neck Pain
2) No foot pain for five weeks
3) Walking with a normal gait
4) Twenty years of chronic knee pain reduced to very minor level, most days pain-free.

Physician (anonymous)
"original main complaint: right mid foot pain, chronic right knee pain and stiffness in gait.
It has been one week since last treatment. Just the slightest hint of stiffness has crept into right foot and knee since yesterday. No other complaint."

Today's treatment experience:
"No sensitivity in feet during treatment, with one exception. Right foot was very reactive in area of transverse colon all the way across to left foot near splenic flexure

reflex just before descending colon. During treatment to that region of the foot, right thigh experienced 'goose flesh' and mild tremor of short duration followed by intense intestinal growling throughout the rest of the treatment (and for about one hour after the treatment)."

"Immediately following treatment my usual deep relaxation was replaced by an energized mental state of very short duration, (twenty minutes). Within one hour of treatment deep fatigue required a ninety minute nap. Awoke refreshed and alert."

"Feet, knee and gait rejuvenated immediately following treatment."

Next treatment:
"My condition at the start of this treatment: I was just starting to recover from four days of viral respiratory infection and feeling rundown. My feet and knees felt good."

"During the treatment both of my feet were tender in the upper mid-foot, which corresponds to the lungs and lymph areas of the body. Very interesting as this area has never been tender prior to this respiratory bug."

"After treatment I did not have my usual feeling of deep relaxation or fatigue, but felt my mental faculties strengthened and more stamina. Doug tells me this often happens after clients have received several treatments, since energy levels in the body have been restored and rest is no longer required. I'm going to miss that mellow feeling."

Menstrual Irregularities Parts 1-4 (Third Person POV)

Woman in early thirties. Overweight, some health problems. Complaining of allergies, irregular menses, possible pre-diabetic conditions.
Treatment #: 1st treatment
Signs during treatment:
1) Very sensitive feet when walking thumbs and fingers with very light acupressure being applied. Client showed EXTREME sensitivity and begged me to use lighter pressure. The only way I could use lighter pressure was to not touch her feet.

Special reflexes that were noticed: (SS stands for sensitivity scale)
1) Toes, neck, uterus, lymphatic, sciatic were all 10+. Everything else was a 7-9.

Symptoms from the client:

- "That was so painful."
- Client reported feeling like I was cutting her skin with my nails while I worked the reflexes or I was cutting her skin with glass.
- Client extremely relaxed when the treatment ended. Took a nap afterwards.
- Reported her feet felt like they were 'walking on air' after the treatment.

Conclusion of first visit:
I've never seen anyone with this much hypersensitivity to almost all her reflexes. She did mention that she has an extremely low threshold of pain. She's not looking forward to treatment, but to the way she'll feel afterwards.

Treatment #: 2nd treatment
Signs during treatment:
1) Showed a marked drop in sensitivity to all her reflexes on only second treatment. Was able to relax during her treatment, mostly.

Special reflexes that were noticed:
1) Hip/sciatic 10+
2) Eyes/ears left foot 10+
3) Bronchial reflex 7
4) Ovaries 10+

Symptoms from the client:
- "I behaved much better didn't I? It didn't hurt as much."
- Client reported numbness when I applied pressure to the top of her large toes.
- Client again extremely relaxed when the treatment ended. Took a nap afterwards.
- Reported again her feet felt like they were 'walking on air' after the treatment.

Conclusion of second visit:
She still has extreme sensitivity in a couple of areas, but none in the rest of her feet. She was able to relax in only one treatment and is now looking forward to next week's treatment instead of conclusion.

Treatment #: 3rd treatment
Signs during treatment:
Pain was on high alert today, with all reflexes being very sensitive. I used very little pressure yet client was experiencing above average pain.

Special reflexes that were noticed:
1) Hip/sciatic 10+
2) Sinus Reflexes on both feet
3) Bronchial/Chest Lung on right foot 7
4) Ovaries/Uterus 10+

Symptoms from the client:
- "I thought this was supposed to not hurt as much, Doug? I still have not had a menstruation cycle in over a year."
- Client still had not had a period as hoped by making visits with me.
- Client again extremely relaxed when the treatment ended.
- Reported again her feet felt like they were 'walking on air' after the treatment. She just loves that feeling.

Conclusion of third visit:
She still has extreme sensitivity in both feet. This is unusual for a third time visit. And still no progress with menstrual cycle. So far the only benefit to this client has been relaxation. Just goes to show reflexology is not an instant cure for client problems. Only time will tell if reflexology (in this case) will assist her body to normalize.

Treatment #: 4th treatment
Signs during treatment:
Pain was mitigated in this visit. I still used very little pressure yet client was experiencing above average pain only in a few areas.

Special reflexes that were noticed:
1) Sinus Reflexes on both feet
2) Ovaries/Uterus 10+

Symptoms from the client:
- "It wasn't as bad as last week. Only very painful in a few areas."
- Client reported that she began her menstrual cycle two days after her last treatment (number 4). This is significant because she has not had a period in over a year!
- Client again extremely relaxed when the treatment ended. Reported again her feet felt like they were 'walking on air' after the treatment. She just loves that feeling.

Conclusion of fourth visit:
She still has extreme sensitivity in both feet but only in a few areas. It is of interest that

one month after her first session, she started menstruating. The other obvious benefit to this client has been relaxation. As her body begins to 'normalize' she will be helped in other areas as well.

Stroke Victim (Third Person POV)

On October 14th, a healthy 51-year-old man suffered a stroke and was in a coma for a number of days and remained in the Cleveland Clinic for 16 days. He received paralysis to the entire right side of his body including loss of speech and all motor skills on the right hemisphere. However, after being transported to Hillside Clinic, therapy began and a painful process of rehabilitation commenced. On the following February, his physical therapists helped restore his speech to the point where he could be understood and a certain amount of motor skills to the right leg and right arm. However, with all the genuine care from physicians and the physical therapist, his progress came to a screeching halt. That's when his physical therapist recommended me. As a reflexologist, I might be able to help him progress further and started seeing him the following September.

Treatment #: 1, 2 & 3
Signs during treatment:
Here's the issues - little to no range-of-motion in his right hand; nor feeling in the tips of this fingers. Little to no range-of-motion in his right foot; unable to move the great toe. Little to no control of the right leg. He wears a leg brace to help stabilize his right foot; which he has no control over. Unable to substantially control the right arm and perform minor functions (like grabbing a zipper on a pair of pants and pulling). Still slurring in his speech.

- When striking the mid-thoracic reflexes of the spine, along with the hip-sciatic reflexes, would cause a chain reaction in the leg that would cause it to flex at the knee (almost 90% and pulling me out of my sitting position), the hamstring, quad muscles to contract and flare (like a cobra's neck) and then muscles in the leg would roll in a wave-like pattern from the calf up to the medial part of the groin muscle. Then his foot would quiver involuntarily for 30-40 seconds as if he had cold chills. Yet he said he felt no pain and was not in control at all of the motion. He seemed thrilled at the prospect of this kind of muscle expansion since he has not had that happen since the day of his stroke.

- Also when working his right hand between the thumb and the first metacarpal bone, again, extreme flexing of the right bicep and a pulling motion towards his chest. It was as if he and I were arm wrestling. He was elated. He had not experienced muscular contractions of this sort since the day of his stroke. His comment to me was that, "With all the electrogesic put on my leg and my arm, it could not cause all the contractions that I'm seeing!"

- By the third treatment, he has sensation in his right fingertips, greater articulation in his thumb and a greater range-of-motion in the entire arm up to the shoulder. He also can move his right foot and the tip of his great toe; he's able to dorsal flex the great toe for the first time since his stroke. As you can imagine, he is happy with the progress of just three treatments, as am I.

Special reflexes that where noticed:
Right foot Hip-sciatic reflex 10+ SS
Right foot Head/neck reflex 7 SS
Right shoulder reflex 7 SS

Symptoms and reaction from the client:
* "That's just incredible! I am so glad to see the muscles in my leg move like that. There's still hope."
* His response from first treatment was soreness in both feet. Second visit, we did both feet and right arm. He had soreness in his right arm, but he had a greater range-of-motion. No other side affects other than sleepiness from the first treatment.
Conclusion of first three visits:
Even though his speech has not improved, progress has been made in both the right foot as regards the great toe, contraction and range-of-motion in right leg, contraction and range-of-motion in right arm and sensation in phalanges of the right hand. He was very surprised at the progress and I have to admit I was as well. Both of us are very hopeful of continued progress from reflexology treatments. His treatments will continue once a week for the duration.

With his permission, he wants us to continue to follow his case in writing for helping us to understand the reflexology theory and put it to scientific understanding. He knows that there is no cure (I believe this also, that there are no cures in life) but keeping the feet healthy will give him the best chance at organic healing.

One thing that can be said to those naysayers of reflexology is, "Try telling this person that reflexology doesn't work and it's just in his head."
He sees his physician and physical therapist weekly.

Chapter 14 - Observations

Painful Feet At Work (Third Person POV)

Woman in her mid 40's in good physical condition yet has pain in her feet from standing at work all day.

Treatment #: 1st treatment
Signs during treatment:
1) Relaxed and in control of her emotions.
2) Positive personality; no signs of depression.
3) No major health problems to this date to speak of.
4) Just sore feet.

Special reflexes that were noticed:
1) Hallux (side of neck) caused patient to thrash her head and have a neck release of some sort. Client seemed very surprised to have that reaction 2 minutes into treatment.
2) Calcium deposits in feet seemed to be minimal at best
3) Adrenals on both feet (7 SS)
4) Hip/sciatic on both feet (9 SS)
5) Thyroid reflex in left great toe (Hallux) (8 SS)

Reaction from the client:
- "I feel like I am floating on air."
- Client experienced a neck release.
- A feeling of euphoria (the 'Buzz' as I like to call it) was present long after the treatment.
- Patient was walking in a disoriented manner for the first six steps (from the reflexology chair), giggling on how wonderful she felt.
Conclusion of first visit:
A much hoped for reaction to a good treatment. This is the way 80% of my clients feel after first treatment.

Observation Articles:

Pain in The Feet After Loved One Dies

Something I have found to be very strange and I thought needed some attention is "Super-Pain" in the feet. Now remember, this phenomenon is with my advanced clients only and those who have seen me several times over the course of many months. This

strange reaction comes in the form of very intense pain all over the feet.
Why is that strange? Because these clients have two things that are very common to them.
1) They had no pain in their previous visits because of having their feet worked free of all congestion.
2) They've just lost a loved one who they were very close to or have received news that a loved one is very sick (such as cancer).

Time and time again, for no other apparent reason a client will come to me and be in agony with the slightest touch to the feet. Only later they will reveal to me that they have just been through a traumatic moment (or someone they love has).

Still doubt the feet have little to do with revealing stress and sickness? My experience has raised interesting questions in both the client and I that may never answered in our lifetime.

The good news is that even though they sit through a reflexology session (perceived as torturous), their feet (and their body) crave the attention in order to dismiss the stressful agony of their emotional life. It is a blessing to see them leave calm, with a slight smile, and a restful gait that helps them face one more day in this world. Naturally, of course.

Infertility Helped by Reflexology Treatments

This is a summary of an infertile woman of seven years finally conceiving after reflexology treatments. I finally received good news from a client who has been childless for seven years after marriage. This client desperately wanted a child because in the Amish religion, in which she belongs, having children is a true blessing of their faith. Without promises or treating for a specific illness, I told her I would do my best to work all the reflexes in order to get circulation back in her feet. The ovary and the uterus reflexes were 10+.

"I tried everything and nothing seems to work ,Doug. I hope reflexology will help!" - said Mary (not her real name).

After five treatments, Mary became pregnant and was beyond ecstatic (as you could imagine). I asked her if she had done anything different? Food, medicine, herbs, or anything? Her reply was "nothing other than the foot treatments".

Well, I am willing to put one on the scorecard for reflexology helping infertility. I guess those who practiced this modality 4,000 years ago knew what they were doing.

Reflexology Helps Hip and Knee Pain

Well, it just goes to show that reflexology charts are not one-size-fits all. I use a very prominent chart in the reflexology field that shows where the reflexes should be. But people are people and they were around before charts. For instance, I worked on a 59-year-old female client yesterday who has had severe hip pain for over six months. Nothing seemed to give her lasting relief so she was advised to see me.

After working her feet for about twenty minutes, the same reflex (10+ in sensitivity) kept stubborn to the end. What reflex was that? It was her knee reflex. Her hip/sciatic reflex was mild in comparison.

The good news is that after that first treatment her hip pain was gone. That's right! One treatment helped her and of course she has rescheduled for further treatments.

****

As a practicing reflexologist you, too, will see many positive outcomes for your clients. Knowing that you're helping people makes practicing worthwhile.

Chapter 14 - Observations

Chapter Fifteen

Business and Ethics

Business and Ethics

The most joyous aspect of reflexology is actually practicing the modality. If you are going into practice yourself, there are less thrilling – but no less important – aspects to acquaint yourself with. These are the business practices and ethical standards you need to be familiar with.

If the best reflexologist in the world does not apply the practical wisdom to be gleaned from this chapter, he would be out-of-practice very quickly.

Scheduling

Scheduling your clients is a very important aspect of the 'business' side of your practice. Nothing will dry up your client list quite like forgetting a client, double-booking appointments, running a treatment short or starting a treatment late because of poor scheduling. I work in a chiropractor's office and in a health food store (as well as do home visits). This calls for three different protocols with regards to scheduling.

At the chiropractor's office, the office manager and receptionists take calls, schedule appointments and collect monies. This means all I have to do is be there; appointments are scheduled every 30 minutes. This allows for enough time to receive the client (although in the chiropractor's office I am supposed to refer to them as 'patients' – standard doctor's office protocol), perform the treatment and give them time to get their shoes on and exit the treatment room so I can sanitize it. The receptionist gives the patients an appointment card as a reminder for their next visit.

At the health food store, I am fortunate to work with a store staff that will schedule appointments over the phone for me. However, scheduling a client I've just treated for a return appointment and receiving the monies fall under my purview. This takes more time, so I schedule these clients every 45 minutes. With this setup, reminder calls 24 hours before the appointment are helpful to stave off missed appointments.

On the occasions that I do home visits, there has to be flexibility on my part because the circumstances are not all the same. I used to attend to only once client in their home for a higher fee but rising gas prices in 2008 put a stop to that. What I do now is offer services for reflexology 'parties' (for lack of a better word as I'd hardly put what I do to be on par with Tupperware or Mary Kay – not that there is anything wrong with those products).

Essentially what that means is this: I go to the homes of clients who can't come to either of my practice locations provided THEY have lined up a minimum of 8 persons for treatment. They will schedule every 30 minutes for me and the monies are given directly to me at the end of each treatment. I've done up to 14 sessions in a 7-hour period like this.

I also charge just a few dollars more per treatment when traveling, but if a host lines up more than one of these 'parties' I will give them a free treatment for their effort AND work on them last so they get the fullest benefit of being able to relax after their treatments. There are people interested in doing it this way, especially those that live quite a distance from you. If they follow my usual recommendation of once-per-month or bi-monthly treatments to follow the initial treatments then that works for both of us.

Fees

You may be wondering, "How much do I charge in fees for my services?" There are some things to consider:

1. Your level of skill
2. Your training
3. Location / cost of doing business
4. What the market will bear
5. What other reflexologists are charging
6. What can you live with?

As you can see there are several factors to consider in making a decision in fees. If you overcharge you will not get any new clients; if you undercharge no one will value your time.

It is commonly known in today's society that there is a fine line in the perception of value-for-money. You may, however, have the desire to do this for free or as a volunteer, which is admirable. Some reflexologists I know simply receive donations based on what people can afford. They may receive a homemade loaf of bread from an elderly woman in exchange for a treatment. Whatever the case, only you can decide what your market will bear.

File System

There are many different filing systems to use, if your practice involves travel to and from different locations, 8" x 5" client cards in an 8" x 5" box will probably be the handiest for you. Standard files for copious notes are fine if you have many clients and need refreshers for each visit AND you are able to practice in one location. While I consider myself to be technically savvy, I don't keep my client information or financials on the computer. It would take too much time for me to update information to computer for each visit for each client. It is probably because I'm dyslexic with poor typing skills.

For me, it's faster to jot notes on a card and the new client is expected to fill out their contact info on the card. One side of the card has columns for dates of each treatment so I can track how many times I've seen them. They're filed in alphabetical order so I can refer to them as needed. However, everyone is different and you may find it to be faster and easier to keep a client database and financial program to track income and print receipts on computer. Admittedly, for marketing purposes, this is easier than what I do, which is manually go through each card and add new clients to a mailing list I keep on my computer.

For income tracking purposes, my daily income is entered on monthly sheets, divided by week. At the end of the month, the total income is entered and my monthly expenses are tracked with it and both are put in their own folder. At the end of the year I gather my twelve folders and do my taxes. It's a pretty simple setup, really. If you're a bit more of an entrepreneur, you may eventually work your way to having an integrated practice with several different modalities. That will mean more clients, more income and more complications. I strongly recommend researching all the requirements needed.

I recommend that you do not sell products in your reflexology practice. It can get you in hot water from both the government and the clientèle. Even though you would NEVER prescribe medicine, it can be construed as such if you sell products with your treatments. It would appear that when you find issues, you look to match that with a product that you believe will aid them and be a complement to your services.

Two things can go wrong: 1) Because you're not a doctor you can't diagnose and cannot discern a true diagnosis from the feet. How would you know, then, what products would benefit the clients 2) You could sell them a product that may cause them to have an adverse reaction to either the medication they're taking or an allergic reaction that would land them in the hospital.

Here's the point: there is little to no liability working on a client's feet, so why increase your liability a thousand-fold involving yourself in selling holistic products? If you want to own a health food store or become a naturopathic doctor and assume the liability of such, then by all means do so. However, if you want to be a reflexologist and stay one, stick to the feet!

Insurances

Insurances may be acquired or recommended through reflexology associations. There are several and googling 'liability insurances for reflexologists' will yield a wealth of information online. The two main types of insurance you may need are **liability** and **worker's compensation** if you have employees or wish to cover yourself. Make sure your search includes the state and local governments business licensing and insurance requirements if any.

Only a handful of states require massage therapy licenses; however in a couple of states like California, while the state itself does not require a massage therapy license, there are certain municipalities in the state that do require this license. Make sure to check in your locality.

Associations

It can be beneficial to join a state or national reflexology association. You can make contacts, further your own education, receive information on insurances, news about new laws that affect your practice as well as ways to increase your client load. There are several and you can, again, utilize the Internet to search on 'state reflexology associations' or 'national reflexology associations'.

At this time, I'm a member of the RAO (Reflexology Association of Ohio) and appreciate that there are hardworking members who work diligently to keep me informed about changes in the laws and keeping us practitioners informed about conferences and new practical information. There is usually an annual fee, but you will probably find it to be worthwhile.

Ethics

Since one of my practicing locales is in a doctor's office, they are required to meet HIPAA (Health Insurance Portability and Accountability Act of 1996) standards for patient privacy. An inspector comes in and makes sure that nothing identifiable can be seen by patients and persons traveling with them that will give them any information about other patients. They are to feel secure that their information will not be exposed to, or shared with, anyone else.

The chiropractor I work with occasionally refers some of his patients to me if he thinks it may help them. Afterwards we may discuss the treatment and I might have to converse with the office manager about the patient, but that is all. I don't share patient information with family and friends. I give them the same level of confidentiality they expect from any doctor.

Although my other practice venue is not a doctor's office, but at a health food store, the same level of professionalism applies. If you find yourself in that situation, it would be prudent to discuss with the store owner / manager and staff about some basic protocols and the HIPAA laws. You may wish to give thought to a 'notice of confidentiality' form from employees.

Some other things to remember: Do not talk about a client with another client unless you feel that the information will help the client you are talking to. In this case, do not mention names or identifiable data. Don't leave information laying around where it can be accessed by unauthorized persons. Lock your file bin and / or laptop when not in use.

If you are a person who has a hard time saying "No" or "I can't talk about that" simply practice saying it with a gentle smile in front of a mirror until it feels natural.

Another aspect is having a professional demeanor. I've already discussed 'looking professional' but in this regard, I'm referring to 'acting professional'. A reflexologist should not flirt with his or her clients or tell off-color jokes. A 'people-pleaser'-type client may laugh with you and may not reschedule because you've made them uncomfortable.

Brusqueness or rudeness are unacceptable as well. If you have a lousy personality, have the humility to work on changing that. If you have few people in your life that want to be around you, ask those few people to share their honest opinion about your people-skills, swallow your pride, LISTEN and make changes that are necessary. Everyone understands the occasional 'bad day' so work on your acting skills because your clients aren't paying you to put up with it and should NEVER have to see it.

A professional, pleasant, somewhat-detached demeanor is important while the client warming up to you. I've had faithful clients that I've seen for years who make me comfortable to be myself around them. However, I always make sure that 'self' doesn't go anywhere near crossing any boundaries. Remember, it is your job to put them at ease, not their job to 'put up with you' to get their feet done. Instruct your employees, if you have any, in this regard as well. In fact, his or her demeanor is just as important, since he or she is the first and last person the client sees!

Reflexologists seem to have an easier time of things than massage therapists do, mainly because reflexology clients do not need to remove any clothing but shoes. Accusation of 'groping' someone's feet inappropriately are unheard of, thankfully.

Of course, in your journey as a reflexologist there will be dream clients and there will be nightmare clients that you will never want to see again. In the classroom setting, I will provide useful tips on how to secure more of the former and discharge more of the latter.

****

In the practice of reflexology there are many aspects to the 'business' of doing it. This chapter is by no means exhaustive, but will definitely give the budding reflexologist guidance in planning how they will operate his or her practice.

Chapter 15 – Business & Ethics

General Terms

Abduction – to turn away from the midline of the body or from an adjacent part or limb.

Adduction – to turn toward the midline of the body or an adjacent part or limb.

Anatomical position – the upright position of the body with the face forward, arms at the side, and the palms facing forward, used as a reference in describing the relation of body parts to one another.

Anterior – situated before or at the front of.

Clavicle Guideline – is an imaginary horizontal line that separates the shoulders and head from the rest of the body.

Cuboid Oblique Guideline – is an imaginary diagonal line that starts at the tuberosity of the fifth metatarsal base at the cuboid notch and goes to the base of the sternum.

Cuboid Transverse Guideline – is an imaginary line running across the foot that separates the lower extremities from the transverse colon to the Hip-Sciatic Guideline.

Distal – the furthest location from a point of reference.

Dominant Reflexes – are the strongest reflexes in the Hierarchal understanding of the Dominant Theory of Reflexology; these reflexes open the way for the striking of Intermedial and Elementary succession.

Dorsal – of, pertaining to, or situated at the back, or dorsum.

Elementary Reflexes – all other reflexes that help normalize the body with no particular order in how these reflexes influence each other.

Hierarchal – the way reflexes influence one another in a descending order.

Hip-Sciatic Guideline – is an imaginary line that separate the lowest region from the rest of the anatomical structure.

Holding Hand – is the hand that supports the foot and gains leverage for the working hand.

Homeostasis – a state of physiological equilibrium or normalization.

Inferior – lower in place of position; situated beneath.

Intermedial Reflexes – important reflexes that, when struck, open and activate healing channels and communication to the elementary reflexes.

Lateral – of or pertaining to the side; situated at, proceeding from, or directed to a side.

Medial – situated in or pertaining to the middle; median.

Planar – flat or level plane.

Plantar – of or pertaining to the sole of the foot.

Posterior – situated behind or at the rear of.

Proximal – the closest location location to a point of reference.

Superior – Situated above; higher in place of position.

Working Hand - is the hand that strikes reflexes, initiates stretching and extension movements.

Index

2330 B.C. - 2

A

abduction wrist stretch – *see 'self-stretching'*
Achilles stretching – *see 'techniques: stretching'*
Achilles tendon – 166, *see also 'tendons of the feet'*
Achilles tendonitis – *see 'conditions of the feet'*
action potentials – 10
adduction wrist stretch – *see 'self-stretching'*
adenoids – 174
adrenaline – *see 'epinephrine'*
adrenals – *see ' intermedial reflex'*
alimentary – 156
alveoli – 153
amygdala – 21, 100-103
amygdala / brain – 100-103
    technique – *see 'techniques'*
anatomy:
    feet, of the – 30
anatomical positional terms:
    abduction -
    adduction -
    anteroposterior – 125
    distal – 57
    dorsal – 57
    lateral – 57
    medial – 57
    plantar – 57
    proximal – 57
Anterior Cruciate Ligament – *see 'ligaments'*
appendix – 164
arches:
    lateral longitudinal – 32
    medial longitudinal – 32
    transverse – 32
arms – 159
arms / hands / elbows / wrist / biceps / triceps – *see 'elementary reflex'*
artery: - 151
    aorta – 151
    pulmonary – 151
arthritis – *see 'conditions of the feet'*
associations – 193
Athlete's foot – *see 'conditions of the feet'*
atria – 151
auditory canal – 149
auditory tube (Eustachian) – 149
auricle – 149
autonomic nervous system – *see 'nervous system'*
axons – 10

B

bad breath – *see 'halitosis'*
basic finger techniques – *see 'techniques'*
biceps – 159
bladder – 161
body members:
    defensive stance – 14, 22
    subservient behavior – 14
bones of the feet:
    diagram – 30
    hallux – 31
    metatarsal – 31
    number of – 30
    phalanges – 31
    tarsals – 32
        calcaneus – 32
        cuboid – 32
        cuneiforms – 32
        navicular – 32
        talus – 32
brachial plexus – *see 'nerve'*
brain – 103
    technique – *see 'techniques'*
breasts – 154
bronchi – 153
bronchial – 153
bronchioles – 153
bronchiolitis – 154
bronchitis - 153
bunions (hallux valgus) – *see 'conditions of the toes'*
business & ethics – 190
buttocks (nates) – 171

C

calcaneus – 166, *see also 'bones of the feet: tarsals'*
calcaneus rocking – *see 'techniques: relaxation'*
calcitonin – 134
calluses – *see 'conditions of the feet'*
carotid artery – 132
cartilage: - 166
    costal – 169
    meniscus:
        lateral – 166
        medial – 166
cecum – *see 'colon'*
cervicals – 121
charts:
    anatomical understanding – 16
    dominant reflex diagram – 62

Index

C *cont'd.*

    Dominant Theory vs. Zone Theory – 16
    guidelines: – 57-58
        clavicle – 57
        cuboid oblique – 57
        cuboid transverse – 58
        hip / sciatic – 58
        intermedial reflex diagram – 63
        medial / lateral view – 61
        plantar view – 60
        spinal misalignments – 124
        traditional – 15
cholesterol – 137
chyme – 140
clavicle guideline – *see 'charts: guidelines'*
clavicles – 168, *see also 'elementary reflex'*
claw toes – *see 'conditions of the toes'*
cleanliness – 69
client communication – 95
client greeting and preparation – 92, 93
club foot – *see 'conditions of the feet'*
cochlea – 149
colognes – 70
colon: – 160
    cecum – 160
    descending – 160
    hepatic flexure – 160
    sigmoid flexure – 161
    splenic flexure – 160
    transverse colon – 160
conditions of the feet:
    Achilles tendonitis – 45
    arthritis – 38
    Athlete's foot – 45
    calluses – 40
    club foot – 46
    corns – 40
    diabetes – 40
    dry skin – 46
    gout – 38
    heel spur - 43
    metatarsalgia - 44
    Morton's neuroma - 44
    neuropathy – 40
    osteoarthritis – 39
    peripheral vascular disease – 41
    plantar fasciitis – 41
    rheumatoid arthritis – 39
    tarsal tunnel syndrome – 39
conditions of the toes:
    bunions (hallux valgus) – 50
    claw toes – 48
    hammer toes – 49
    ingrown toenails (onychocrytosis) – 53
    mallet toes – 49
    Morton's Toe – 50
    toenail fungus (onychomychosis) – 52
    webbed toes (syndactyly) – 51
congestion – 11, 15, 21
    real (calcium & uric acid) – 18
    types of – 24
COPD – 154
cornea – 148
corns – *see 'conditions of the feet'*
cortex – 137
cortisol – 138
cortisone – 137
cuboid – *see 'bones of the feet: tarsals'*
cuboid oblique guideline – *see 'charts: guidelines'*
cuboid transverse guideline – *see 'charts: guidelines'*
cuneiforms – *see 'bones of the feet: tarsals'*

D

deltoids – *see 'elementary reflex'*
dermis – 7
descending colon – *see 'colon'*
diabetes – *see 'conditions of the feet'*
diagnose: – 14, 15, 23, 146
    client communication – 25
    traditional charts – 15
diagnostic:
    internal – 13, 15
digital dorsal flexion – *see 'techniques: stretching'*
distal – *see 'anatomical positional terms'*
dominant reflex: - 18, 19
    amygdala / brain – 100-103
        technique – *see 'techniques'*
    hip / sciatic – 116-117
        technique – *see 'techniques'*
    hypothalamus / pituitary / pineal – 106-108
        technique – *see 'techniques'*
    opens – 12
    spine – 121-122
        technique – *see 'techniques'*
    table of reflexes – 20
    trapezius shoulders – 110-111
        technique – *see 'techniques'*
Dominant Theory – 4, 16, 18
dorsal – *see 'anatomical positional terms'*
dorsal digits down – *see 'techniques: trapezius shoulders'*
dorsal hand flex – *see 'self-stretching'*
dry skin – *see 'conditions of the feet'*
duodenum – 139, 156, 160

Index

E

ears – 148
electrolyte – 137
elementary reflex: - 18, 19, 146
    arms / hands / elbows / wrist / biceps / triceps – 159
        technique – *see 'techniques'*
    deltoids – 155
        technique – *see 'techniques'*
    gallbladder – 158
        technique – *see 'techniques'*
    gluteus maximus / low back – 171
        technique – *see 'techniques'*
    heart / pectoralis major / ribs / esophagus / bronchials / breasts – 151-154
        technique – *see ' techniques'*
    ileocecal valve / appendix – 164
        technique – *see 'techniques'*
    latissimus dorsi – 170
        technique – *see 'techniques'*
    legs / knees / Achilles tendons / gastrocnemius / hamstrings / quadriceps – 165
    sinus / head / eyes / ears – 147-150
        technique – *see 'techniques'*
    small intestine / colon / bladder / ureters / testes / ovaries / uterus / prostate – 160
        technique – *see 'techniques'*
    spleen – 158
        technique – *see 'techniques'*
    stomach – 156
        technique – *see 'techniques'*
    table of reflexes – 20
endocrine – 21, 135, 139
epicranius – *see 'muscles'*
epidermis – 7
epinephrine (adrenaline) – 137
equipment – 70
esophagus – 153
estrogen – 162
ethics – 194
exocrine – 139
eyes – 148

F

fascia – 30, 43
fees – 191
femur – 165
fibula – 165
file system – 192
Fitzgerald, Dr. William – 2
flexor hallicus longus – *see 'tendons of the feet'*
frontalis – *see 'muscles'*

G

galea – 130
gallbladder – *see 'elementary reflex'*
gastrocnemius – 35, 166-167
gladiolus (body) – 169
glucagon – 139
glucose – 139
gluteus maximus / low back – 171, *see also 'elementary reflex'*
gout – *see 'conditions of the feet'*

H

halitosis (bad breath) – 69
hallux – *see 'bones of the feet'*
hallux valgus (bunions) – *see 'conditions of the toes'*
hammer toes – *see 'conditions of the toes'*
hamstrings – 167
hand drill – *see 'techniques: relaxation'*
hands – 159
hanging the saddle – *see 'techniques: relaxation'*
head – 147
heart – 151-152
heel spurs – *see 'conditions of the feet'*
hepatic flexure – *see 'colon'*
Hierarchal – 4, 18
hip / sciatic guideline – *see 'charts: guidelines'*
histamine – 164
holding techniques – *see 'techniques'*
holistic – 25
Holland Method of Advanced Reflexology – 4, 6-7
homeostasis:
    checks and balances – 13
    feet, body's designate – 12
humerus – 152
hydrochloric acid – 156
hyperthyroidism – 134
hypothalamus – 21, 22, 106
    technique – *see 'techniques'*
hypothyroidism – 135

I

ileocecal valve – 160, 164
ileum – 160
illustrations:
    massage therapists – 19
    pain, why do reflexes hurt – 9
    paralyzed, severed spine – 13
    psychologist – 12
    reflex, striking a – 9

I *cont'd.*

    rock in the shoe – 22
    sewing machine – 8
immune system – *see 'lymphatic system'*
incus – 149
ingesta – 161
Ingham, Eunice – 3
ingrown toenails (onychocryptosis) – *see 'conditions of the toes'*
insulin – 139
insurances – 193
intent statement – 94
intermedial reflex: - 18, 19, 130
    adrenals – 137-138
        technique – *see 'techniques'*
    kidneys – 143-144
        technique – *see 'techniques'*
    liver – 141
        technique – *see 'techniques'*
    occipitalis – 130
        technique – *see 'techniques'*
    pancreas – 139
        technique – *see 'techniques'*
    sternocleidomastoid / neck – 132
        technique – *see 'techniques'*
    table of reflexes – 20
    thyroid / parathyroids – 134-135
        technique – *see 'techniques'*
interphalangeal – *see 'joints'*
islets of langerhans – 139

J

jejunum – 140, 160
joints:
    feet, of the – 31
    interphalangeal – 31
        distal – 31
        proximal – 31
    metatarsointerphalangeal joint – 132
    metatarsophalangeal – 31
    popping – 31

K

kidneys – *see 'intermedial reflex'*
kidney stones – 144
knees – 165

L

labyrinth – 149
lactic acid – 141
lateral – *see 'anatomical positional terms'*
Lateral Collateral Ligament – *see 'ligaments'*
latissimus dorsi – 170
legs – 165
lens – 148
levels of pressure – *see 'techniques'*
leverage – *see 'techniques'*
liability – *see 'insurances'*
ligaments: - 166
    Anterior Cruciate – 166
    Lateral Collateral – 166
    Medial Collateral – 166
    Posterior Cruciate – 166
lighting – 71
liver – *see 'intermedial reflex'*
low back – *see 'gluteus maximus'*
lumbars – 121
lymphatic system – 174
lymphocytes – 174-175

M

macrophages – 175
mallet toes – *see 'conditions of the toes'*
malleus – 149
manubrium – 169
medial – *see 'anatomical positional terms'*
Medial Collateral Ligament – *see 'ligaments'*
medulla – 137
metatarsal – *see 'bones of the feet'*
metatarsal stretching – *see 'techniques: stretching'*
    abduction – *see 'techniques: stretching: metatarsal'*
    adduction – *see 'techniques: stretching: metatarsal'*
    wrenching – *see 'techniques: stretching: metatarsal'*
metatarsal wave – *see 'techniques: relaxation'*
metatarsalgia – *see 'conditions of the feet'*
metatarsointerphalangeal joint – *see 'joints'*
metatarsophalangeal – *see 'joints'*
Morton's neuroma – *see 'conditions of the feet'*
Morton's Toe – *see 'conditions of the toes'*
mucosa – 140
muscles:
    epicranius – 130
    deltoids – *see 'elementary reflex'*
    frontalis – 130
    occiptalis – 130
muscles of the feet:
    flexor digitorum brevis – 34
    flexor hallicus brevis – 34

Index

M *cont'd.*

music – 71

N

nail care – 68
nates (buttocks) – 171
navicular – *see 'bones of the feet: tarsals'*
nephron – 143
nerve:
    brachial plexus – 132
    cells – 11
    cranial – 122
    impulses – 10
    feet, of the – 35
    pain – 12
    peripheral – 122
    spinal – 122
nervous system:
    autonomic – 21
    parasympathetic – 21, 22
    peripheral -
    sympathetic – 21, 22
neuropathy – *see 'conditions of the feet'*
nodal – 148
norepinephrine – 137

O

observation – 15
observations & experiences: 178
    help with hip and knee pain – 187
    help with infertility – 186
    pain in feet after death of loved one – 185
    physician – 178
    stroke victim – 183
    woman (30's) – 180
    woman (40's) – 185
occipitalis – 130
    technique – *see 'techniques'*
oils and lotions – 96
onychocryptosis (ingrown toenail) – *see 'conditions of the toes'*
onychomychosis (toenail fungus) – *see 'conditions of the toes'*
orthotics – 33
osteoarthritis – *see 'conditions of the feet'*
ovaries – 162

P

pain: – 17
    contradictions in – 18
'pain and observation' – 10
pancreas – *see 'intermedial reflex'*
parasympathetic nervous system – *see 'nervous system'*
parathyroids – *see 'intermedial reflex'*
patella – 165
pectoralis major – 152
peripheral nervous system – *see 'nervous system'*
peripheral vascular disease – *see 'conditions of the feet'*
peristalsis – 153
phalanges – *see 'bones of the feet'*
phalanges exercise – *see 'self-stretching'*
pharynx – 153
pineal gland – 108
    technique – *see 'techniques'*
pituitary – 17, 107
    technique – *see 'techniques'*
planar – 34
plantar – *see 'anatomical positional terms'*
plantar digits down – *see 'techniques: trapezius shoulders'*
plantar digits up – *see 'techniques: trapezius shoulders'*
plantar fasciitis – *see 'conditions of the feet'*
plantar hand flex – *see 'self-stretching'*
Posterior Cruciate Ligament – *see 'ligaments'*
progesterone – 162
pronation – 33
prostate – 161
proximal – *see 'anatomical positional terms'*
pupil – 148

Q

quadriceps - 167

R

record-keeping – 92
reflex: – 7
    Dominant Theory – 16
    powerful reaction – 12
    striking a – 11
    table of – 20

reflexology, definition of – 6
relaxation – *see 'techniques'*
retina – 148
rheumatoid arthritis – *see 'conditions of the feet'*
ribs: – 152

Index

R *cont'd.*
    false – 152
    floating – 152
    true – 152

S

sacculus – 149
sacral / coccyx – 121
sacroiliac joint – 116
scapular depression – 111
scapular elevation – 111
scapular retraction – 111
scheduling – 190
sciatica – 116
self-stretching: – 66-68
    abduction wrist stretch – 67
    adduction wrist stretch – 67
    dorsal hand flex – 66
    phalanges exercise – 68
    plantar hand flex – 67
sigmoid flexure – *see 'colon'*
sinus / head / eyes / ears – *see 'elementary reflex'*
sinuses: 147
    ethmoid – 147
    frontal – 147
    maxillary – 147
    paranasal – 147
    sphenoid – 147
skin – 7
small intestine – *see 'elementary reflex'*
small intestine / colon / bladder / ureters / testes /
    ovaries / uterus / prostate – *see 'elementary reflex'*
spine – 121-125
    technique – *see 'techniques'*
spleen – 174, *see also 'elementary reflex'*
splenic flexure – *see 'colon'*
stapes – 149
sternocleidomastoid – 59, 132
sternocleidomastoid / neck – *see 'intermedial reflex'*
    technique – *see 'techniques'*
sternum – 169, *see also 'elementary reflex'*
stomach – *see 'elementary reflex'*
stretching techniques – *see 'techniques'*
subcutis – 7
supination – 34
syndactyly (webbed toes) – *see 'conditions of the toes'*
sympathetic nervous system – *see 'nervous system'*

T

table of reflexes – 20
talus – *see 'bones of the feet: tarsals'*
tarsals – *see 'bones of the feet'*
tarsal stretching – *see 'techniques: stretching'*
tarsal tunnel syndrome – *see 'conditions of the feet'*
techniques:
    adrenals – 138
    amygdala / brain – 103-105
    arms / hands / elbows / wrist / biceps / triceps – 159
    basic finger – 75
    clavicles – 168
    deltoids – 155
    gallbladder – 158
    gluteus maximus / low back – 171
    heart / pectoralis major / ribs / esophagus /
        bronchials / breasts – 154
    hip / sciatic – 118-120
        lateral compression and extension – 118
        lateral finger drive – 119
        medial compression and extension – 118
        medial finger drive – 119
    holding – 80
    hypothalamus / pituitary / pineal – 109
    ileocecal valve / appendix – 164
    latissimus dorsi – 170
    legs / knees / Achilles tendons / gastrocnemius /
        hamstrings / quadriceps – 167
    levels of pressure – 77
        level one – 77
        level two – 77
        level three – 78
    leverage – 79
    liver – 142
    occipitalis – 131
    pancreas – 140
    relaxation: -
        calcaneus rocking – 85
        hand drill – 86
        hanging the saddle – 88
        metatarsal wave – 87
    sinus / head / eyes / ears – 150
    small intestine / colon / bladder / ureters / testes /
        ovaries / uterus / prostate – 163
    spine – 125-126
    spleen – 158
    sternocleidomastoid / neck – 132-133
    sternum – 169
    stomach – 156
    stretching – 80
        Achilles – 84
        digital dorsal flexion – 84

T *cont'd.*

    metatarsal – 81
        abduction – 82
        adduction – 82
        wrenching – 82-83
    tarsal – 80
    thyroid / parathyroids – 136
    trapezius shoulders – 112
        dorsal digits down – 115
        plantar digits down – 114
        plantar digits up – 114
        walking the ridge – 112

tendons of the feet:
    Achilles – 35
    flexor hallicus longus – 35
testes – 161
thoracics – 121
thumb-driving (walking) – 8, 74
thymus – 174
thyroid – 22, 134-135 (*see also 'intermedial reflex'*)
tibia – 165
toenail fungus (onychomychosis) – *see 'conditions of the toes'*
tonsils – 174
touch vs. tools – 14
transverse colon – *see 'colon'*
trapezius shoulders – 110-111
treatment:
    beginning – 96
    length – 76
triceps – 159
tryptophan – 164

U

uric acid – 18, 30
ureters – 161
uterus – 162
utriculus – 149

V

veins (vena cava) 151
ventricles – 151
vertebra(e) – 121
vertebral canal – 122
vestibule – 149
vitreous humor – 148

W

webbed toes (syndactyly) – *see 'conditions of the toes'*
walking the ridge – *see 'techniques: trapezius shoulders'*
worker's compensation – see 'insurances'

X

xiphoid process – 169

Z

Zone Therapy – 2, 16, 18

Index

Bibliography

Byers, Dwight C.; <u>Better Health with Foot Reflexology</u>. Ingham Publishing, 2000. Pgs. 3-6 History of Reflexology.

Clarkson, Hazel M.; <u>Musculoskeletal Assessment: Joint Range of Motion and Manual Muscle Strength.</u> Lippincott Williams & Wilkins, 1999. Pgs. 138-139.

Dougans, Inge and Ellis, Suzanne; <u>The Art of Reflexology</u>. Element Books, Inc., 1992. Pgs. 11-14 History of Reflexology.

Gray, Henry; <u>Anatomy of the Human Body</u>. Lea & Febiger, 1918. Illustrations.

Johnson, Leonard R. and John H. Byrne; <u>Essential Medical Physiology.</u> Academic Press, 2003. Pgs. 72-75.

Wills, Pauline; <u>The Reflexology Manual</u>. Healing Arts Press, 1995. Pgs. 8-10 History of Reflexology.

About The Author

Douglas Richard Holland, Jr. was born in 1968 in Plentywood, Montana. He was raised in Southwest Florida to adulthood and has been married to Lori since 1991. They have two children, Bouldin (1995) and Paige (1998).

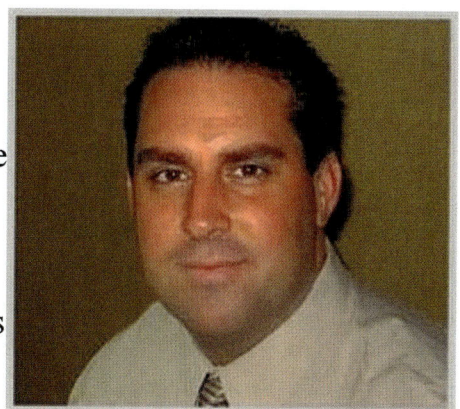

Doug began his reflexology career after being certified from the International Institute of Reflexology as well as becoming certified as an Advanced Integrative Reflexologist at the Advanced Integrative Medical Institute in Washington DC in 2001.

He has practiced his modality in Highlands-Cashiers, NC; Bozeman, Montana and recently in Northeastern Ohio where he has close to a thousand clients in his two practicing locales. He has opened the minds of many professionals in the allopathic health field and many have become his staunchest advocates.

Unfortunately, there is not enough reflexologists in the Midwest to educate and handle the demand of individuals who truly need this modality.

It was his desire to make sure more people could receive the benefits of reflexology and that is why he has opened the Holland Institute of Reflexology; to teach his method to a new generation of reflexologists. He also decided that a book geared for his students, yet practical for the general public could be used as a tool to educate individuals on how to perform reflexology.

Doug enjoys working and relaxing with his family. In his off time he likes researching, fishing, hunting, working out, wine-making, mountain-biking, snowboarding and four-wheeling.

Made in the USA
Monee, IL
03 August 2023